Provided as a service to
medicine by AstraZeneca

T

A practical introduction

Edited by
Deborah Kirklin
and Ruth Richardson

Royal College of Physicians
of London

Publisher's acknowledgement

The Royal College of Physicians is pleased to acknowledge generous educational grants from **Pfizer Ltd** and **The Cancer Research Campaign** towards the production costs of this book.

Front cover

The cover for this book features a painting by Michele Petrone entitled *The Maze of Trees*. Faced with the fear and uncertainty posed by a serious illness, Michele searched for a path ahead.

Royal College of Physicians of London
11 St Andrews Place, London NW1 4LE.

Registered Charity No. 210508

Copyright © 2001 Royal College of Physicians of London

ISBN 1 86016 147 2

A catalogue record of this book is available from the British Library

Designed by Merriton Sharp, London
Printed in Great Britain by Sarum Print Limited, Salisbury, Wiltshire

Contents

Contributors

The contributors to this book are active in pioneering the delivery of medical humanities across the United Kingdom. A number of them are associated with the Medical Humanities Unit based with the Department of Primary Care and Population Sciences at the Royal Free and University College Medical School. This will hereafter be referred to as the Medical Humanities Unit.

Heather Allan – a psychotherapist – is a tutor at the Medical Humanities Unit.

Phil Barker – a nurse – is Professor of Psychiatric Nursing at Newcastle University.

Michael Baum – a surgeon – is Emeritus Professor of Surgery, Visiting Professor of Medical Humanities at the Royal Free and University College Medical School, and a member of the Medical Humanities Unit Steering Group.

Gillie Bolton – a writer – is a Medical Humanities Research Associate at Sheffield Medical School and a member of the Medical Humanities Unit Steering Group.

Mobasher Butt, **Ellie Cannon** and **Sinead Doherty** are writers. They are also medical students at the Royal Free and University College Medical School.

Martyn Evans – a philosopher – is a Senior Lecturer at the University of Wales School of Medicine, Swansea, and co-editor of the journal *Medical Humanities*.

Jonathan Glover – a philosopher – is Professor of Medical Law and Ethics at the Centre for Medical Law and Ethics, King's College, London.

Wendy Hughes – a writer – is a tutor at the Medical Humanities Unit.

Brian Hurwitz – a general practitioner – is Professor of Primary Health Care and General Practice, Imperial College of Science, Technology & Medicine, London.

Deborah Kirklin – a general practitioner – is a Lecturer in Medical Humanities at the Royal Free and University College Medical School, and Co-Director of the Medical Humanities Unit.

John Wyn Owen – a policy-maker – is the Secretary of the Nuffield Trust.

Michele Angelo Petrone – an artist – is a tutor at the Medical Humanities Unit.

Ruth Richardson – an inter-disciplinary historian – is a Research Associate at the Medical Humanities Unit and at the Wellcome Trust Centre for the History of Medicine, University College, London.

Foreword

Professor Sir David Weatherall FRS
Regius Professor of Medicine, University of Oxford

A few years ago the editor of the *British Medical Journal* asked me to write an editorial for the Christmas edition based on a series of articles that he was publishing, written by patients who had had a variety of bad experiences, all of which stemmed from the uncaring attitudes and lack of sensitivity of their doctors.[1] In searching for an explanation for these horror stories I discussed the more obvious problems for present day doctors, including the frenetic pace of modern, high-technology medicine, adding that it is possible that at least some of the shortcomings of current clinical care stem from our education system in general, and medical education in particular. I pointed out that young people, if they wish to become doctors, have to specialise in science at school from the age of fifteen, then spend five or six years trying to cope with the overcrowded curricula of their medical schools, after which they are thrown into the frenetic hothouse of modern hospital life. It is no wonder that they never have the time to learn enough about the world to be able to ponder the multi-faceted problems of sick people.

After the article was published I had the most extraordinary series of letters from all over the world, a few supportive but the majority ranging from highly critical to frankly abusive. It was clear that, if nothing else, many of my colleagues consider themselves to be extremely well-rounded human beings!

No doubt my rather desperate attempts to explain the basis for the sad stories recounted by these patients was inadequate. However, as somebody who has been teaching and practising medicine for over forty years, I still find it difficult to explain why these things happen. It seems to me that young people who are entering medical school these days are much more caring than those of my generation. Indeed, some of the attitudes and approaches to patient care that I observed in my teachers would never be tolerated today. Perhaps the profession has never really got it right, and we have only become aware of our shortcomings in recent years as society has become much more demanding of its doctors. But whatever the reason, the horror stories continue, and a day rarely goes by without some grizzly tale about the inadequacies of medical care in this country.

Given such a bad press it is not surprising that medical education has been experiencing a period of intense self-examination. The traditional Western methods of training doctors based on the lines of Flexner[2] and others are being abandoned. Students are being encouraged to interact with patients right from the beginning of their training, the teaching of basic biological sciences is being diluted with much more emphasis on the social sciences, ethics, communication skills and the many other facets of training which are deemed to be needed to develop the humane, pastoral and communicative skills required of a good doctor.

Many of those who would reform medical education believe that a genuine understanding of the human condition can be gained only through introducing studies of the arts and humanities into the curriculum. This, they argue, is the only way that the medical ethos can be humanised from its current mechanistic and inward looking state. For example, the General Medical Council has recommended, if that is a strong enough word, that medical schools introduce special study modules which will expose students to literature, arts, and other subjects completely outside the usual run of a medical curriculum.[3] The Council is even asking that these modules are assessed, and in exactly the same way as the rest of the course. This new angle on the education of doctors of the future has become a major issue in many medical schools and is developing a life of its own.

To what extent are we justified in adding yet another series of hurdles to an overcrowded medical curriculum, particularly at a time when medical schools are being asked to reduce the amount of taught material and to give students more time to work on their own and to think? Few would doubt the value of a good background in the humanities as at least one facet needed to encourage the broad understanding of the human condition required of doctors. On the other hand, the introduction of the humanities as an examined part of the curriculum does have the feel of a remedial exercise, which is making up for the deficiences of our national education system. If this were broader based, and young people were not encouraged to specialise in science so early if they wish to become doctors, they would have a much wider appreciation of the humanities and would come to enjoy them for what they are; it would then be unnecessary to teach them more formally in this way.

This new trend raises an even broader issue. Is it possible for young people, having had a rather narrow education and who entered medical school very young, to have experienced enough of the world to be able to appreciate the insights into what makes us what we are that can be found in great works of literature or fine art? Shouldn't we be focussing our efforts on trying to increase the breadth of education in our schools and, at the same time, encourage youngsters who wish to become doctors to spend some time travelling and working in other fields before they enter medical school, so that they have a better appreciation of their fellow human beings?

I only voice these concerns in introducing this fine book on medical education and the humanities in the sincere hope that, in our genuine wish to produce more rounded doctors and to comply with the requirements of bodies that oversee medical education, we will not move towards a state of national uniformity in medical education. Rather we must go on thinking about how best to achieve our aims, for a profession as wonderful and diverse as medicine must continue to offer diversity in the training of those who wish to become doctors. But the movement started by those who wish to integrate teaching of the humanities into the medical curriculum must certainly be explored, and this excellent book will provide a great deal of help and inspiration to those who are moving in this direction.

The editors have brought together a splendid team of writers of diverse backgrounds who bring a great deal of wisdom and experience to help readers develop programmes to teach the humanities in a clinical setting. It is difficult to imagine that the kind of approaches that are outlined in these broad-based chapters will not go at least some way to widening students' horizons and, perhaps even more importantly, they might help to generate a level of humility which is so often lacking in our profession and which is, I suspect,the basis for many of its shortcomings.

In a recent editorial on the humanities as special study modules, one of the editors of this book introduced the topic with a quotation from Checkov: '... the sensitivity of the artist may equal the knowledge of the scientist. Both have the same object, nature, and perhaps in time it will be possible for them to link together in a great and marvellous force which is at present hard to imagine'[4]. This seems to go to the heart of what these new movements in medical education should be all about.

The long-standing debate between CP Snow (scientist and novelist) and FR Leavis (literary critic) about the 'two cultures' was surely one of the most sterile exercises ever embarked on[5]. There is no fundamental difference between the aspirations of the great artist and the great scientist or, for that matter, the great clinician. They are all striving to explore nature, or human nature, and understand its complexities for what they are.

The approach taken by this book is, happily, integrative rather than divisive; if presented in this way this new aspect of medical education can only do good. As I have emphasised, it is only one approach to solving our problems, and could become less important if our education system becomes more broad-based. But since this may not happen for a very long time, if ever, we may be stuck with trying to make up for the deficiencies of the educational breadth of young people entering medical school for a while to come.

It is always a delight to be invited to produce a foreword to a book that is being written or edited by one of one's former students. If nothing else, it is reassuring to discover that, despite our bungling efforts to teach medical students, a few of them escape unscathed. Indeed, when I look at the quality of young people coming into medical schools these days I rest happy with the thought that it would take a better man than me to damage them permanently.

March 2001   DW

Notes and references

1 Weatherall D. The inhumanity of medicine. *BMJ* 1994;**309**:1671-1672 (24 December).

2 Abraham Flexner's Report, Medical Education in the United States and Canada, published in 1910 as Bulletin No. 4 of the Carnegie Foundation for the Advancement of Education, revolutionised medical education in the USA and elsewhere, stressing the importance of a sound scientific base.

3 General Medical Council. *Tomorrow's doctors: recommendations on undergraduate medical education.* London: General Medical Council, 1993.

4 Checkov A. Draft of a letter to Gregorovitch. In: Coope J. *Doctor Checkov: a study in literature and medicine.* Isle of Wight: Cross Publishing, 1997.

5 Based on CP Snow's Rede Lecture, 'The two cultures and the scientific revolution', given in 1959 in Cambridge. His views were strongly attacked by FR Leavis in the *Times Literary Supplement*, 23rd April, 1970.

A message from the President of the Royal College of Physicians

The following sentence, taken from the first chapter of this book, expresses well the role that the humanities can play in educating and supporting humanistic physicians and why this is needed now more than ever.

At a time when the medical profession finds its culture, traditions and systems of self-regulation under increasing scrutiny, medical humanities can create a welcome and necessary space to acknowledge the conflicting demands and stresses that are part and parcel of our working lives, to examine the driving force behind our practice and to connect through our shared humanity with the individuals who entrust themselves to our care.

The pressure on today's doctors starts at medical school with its crowded curriculum. It grows as they progress through their careers and have to assimilate the ever proliferating medical advances while striving to manage increasing workloads – often with less than adequate facilities and support, and often under the harsh spotlight of media and public scrutiny. This leaves them but little time for reflection and can engender a mechanistic approach to medical practice. But medicine is a caring profession, requiring sensitivity and imagination. However sound their medical knowledge, doctors who do not have these attributes do not make good clinicians. The study of the humanities – art , creative writing, poetry, philosophy, to name but a few of the subjects that come within its broad remit – through stimulating their imagination and providing time for thought will enable medical students, doctors and indeed all health care professionals to gain better insight into their own motivation and practice. Just as importantly, of course, it will help them to empathise and deal sensitively with patients and their families when they are often at their most vulnerable and in need of understanding.

I wholeheartedly endorse the ideas behind this timely book. It is entirely appropriate that this College should publish it and we are pleased to do so.

March 2001   KGMM Alberti
                                   President, Royal College of Physicians

Editors' preface

Medical humanities, interpreted very broadly, can be held to encompass any interaction between the arts and health: a field rich in potential. Our intention here is modest, the focus being the role of the humanities in medical education.

Arts-informed medical education is currently experiencing a renaissance, both in popularity and acceptability. The aim here is to offer encouragement and practical assistance to all those interested in this field, providing an introduction and overview to help those wishing to integrate medical humanities into their own teaching, and learning. It is aimed at all those interested or involved in the education, training, mentoring and support of health care professionals of every discipline.

This book does not claim to be either the first or the last word on this subject, but we hope that this practical introduction to medical humanities will offer not only ideas, inspiration and reference to good practice from around the country, but also renewed enthusiasm. We believe the innovations in medical education described here will be of great interest to patients, and to those active in using the arts to improve health and well-being. The book concludes with a guide to further reading, drawn from suggestions by our authors.

Acknowledgements

Our first thanks must go to each of the contributors who have worked so hard to make this book possible, and to Diana Beaven, Andrew Lamb and Peter Watkins at the Royal College of Physicians for their enthusiasm in bringing this volume to press.

The national conference, 'The healing arts: the role of the humanities in medical education', which laid the foundation for a number of chapters in this volume, was held on the 30th March 2000. It was supported by educational grants from Pfizer Limited, The Nuffield Trust and The Cancer Research Campaign, and was hosted by the Royal Society of Arts.

We are indebted to Dr Richard Meakin, Dr Margaret Lloyd, Dr Surinder Singh, Sophie Parker and Heather Mitchell for their help throughout this project and to Professor Robin Downie, Dr Trish Greenhalgh and Susan Loppert for their reading suggestions.

Dedication

We dedicate this book to all those patients, artists, writers, students and fellow tutors who have shared their stories, dreams and imaginings with us, and to our spouses, Kelley Kirklin and Brian Hurwitz, in grateful recognition of their tolerance, patience and humanity.

Deborah Kirklin
Ruth Richardson

Medical humanities and tomorrow's doctors

There is, of course, nothing new about the idea that the arts can play a valuable role in the education of health care professionals.[1] The ancients conceived medicine as a fundamental branch of philosophy. To Hippocrates, medicine is an art. Only by close and careful observation of the patient can the doctor hope to be successful.[2] It is only in relatively recent times that the professional and public perception of medicine has shifted to a biomedical model: the dominant impression that the practice of medicine is governed by scientific truths subject, at least in theory, to experimental verification. So it is perhaps timely to remember that philosophy (the love of wisdom) underpins all scientific endeavour.

The publication of *Tomorrow's doctors*[3] by the education committee of the General Medical Council (GMC) in 1993 marked a turning point for those who, like Professor Robin Downie and Professor Sir Kenneth Calman, have been championing the developing discipline of medical humanities for many years.[4]

Tomorrow's doctors called on, and indeed required, all medical schools in the UK to implement radical changes to the undergraduate medical curriculum: crucially the document proposed the introduction of a core medical school syllabus, and the suggested allocation of up to thirty percent of the timetable to optional 'special study modules' (SSMs).[5] The possibility of arts-based courses within these modules was highlighted by the GMC, which cited the appropriateness of courses such as Literature and Medicine.

It is not yet known how many medical schools have taken up this option, or how many students have taken advantage of arts-based SSMs. However, reports of courses are beginning to be published and it is clear that medical educators are taking advantage of the opportunity provided by *Tomorrow's doctors* in novel and imaginative ways.[6,7,8] A survey of all SSMs being offered throughout UK medical schools is currently underway, the results of which will be available shortly.[9] Preliminary findings are that incorporation of the humanities into the under-graduate curriculum is already widespread, and that students value it, perceiving it as an attractive option. The value placed by experienced practitioners on an education enriched by the humanities is examined here in chapters 5 and 8. However, enquiries received at our Medical Humanities Unit, at the Royal Free Hospital, suggest that transforming good ideas and enthusiasm into successful, accepted and viable courses can still present quite a challenge. In some medical schools it is still, sadly, true that humanities SSMs are not encouraged. At others the paucity of humanities courses reflects financial constraints, rather than any lack of enthusiasm and expertise. With SSMs set to occupy between ten and thirty percent of the timetable, the question of appropriate funding still needs to be addressed.

Educational objectives

Whilst the concept that the practice of medicine is an art is generally accepted, and whilst an appreciation of the arts comes easily to many doctors, an understanding of what exactly medical humanities seeks to achieve is perhaps harder for many practitioners to define. This question is addressed in chapter 1 by the presentation of four cases of medical humanities 'in action'. Two objectives are outlined. The first is to enable reflective practice, which is explored in greater depth in chapter 8. The second objective is to enable students of all ages better to understand the experiences, perspectives and needs of their patients. With the medical profession under attack for being out of touch with what society expects,[10] the potential of the humanities to help in strengthening the human bonds between doctor and patient ought to be embraced.

An inter-disciplinary field

One of the great strengths and pleasures of medical humanities is the multi-disciplinary collaborations and working partnerships it can involve. This volume brings together the experience and ideas of a range of disciplines, including medicine, philosophy, nursing, psychotherapy, medical history, literature and health policy, as well as the invaluable insights of patients. The editors between them draw on their combined experience as scholars and teachers in medical humanities, medical ethics and law, history of medicine, and communications skills, as well as their experience as doctors, patients, and mothers and kin to patients. Inter-disciplinary collaborations of this type, in a field with exciting and unexplored boundaries, present challenges as well as opportunities. Recognition of the extent, and the limits, of personal and professional competence is central to any success achieved by any single discipline. Appreciating these limitations is essential if doctors are to win the respect of colleagues in the humanities.[11]

Good communication between members of the teaching team, and recognition of the strengths and the weaknesses of the various team members, are therefore crucial. In this way not only will our students receive the learning experience they deserve, but tutors will learn from each other. Cross-fertilisation of insights and perspectives may perhaps lead to novel ways of understanding the very nature of medical endeavour.[12]

The role of the humanities in medical education

The scientific paradigm has hitherto served medicine well, and continues to do so. With an already overcrowded curriculum it is therefore reasonable to ask what incorporating the humanities into the education of health care professionals will add. One answer to this question is given in chapter 3, where examples from literature and art are used to convey the importance of the use of metaphor in understanding the experience of illness. The use of metaphor is integral to the ability of individuals to express the feelings and emotions for which not even a language as rich as English always has words. The value placed by doctors and patients alike on this means of expression and insight is, perhaps, one of the reasons medical humanities has found so many supporters. As the journalist Martyn Harris wrote:

> The frisson you get from a fine line of poetry comes chiefly, I think, from the sheer pleasure that someone has recorded something you thought only you had felt before. More than that, it comes from the realisation that many others have shared and will share with you this moment that you had thought was unique and inexpressible. The loneliness of the individual life is dissolved briefly in the flicker of that same sensation, of coherence.[13]

Martyn Harris's own metaphor expresses well why reading poetry has value. His emphasis on coherence reflects a clear awareness of our shared humanity.

Patient perspectives

It could perhaps be argued that whilst doctors may enjoy participating in and teaching these courses, patients might prefer their doctors to concentrate on honing their diagnostic and technical skills. The point is well taken. But anyone who thinks these skills are sufficient to satisfy all patient needs should read the perspectives provided by Michele Petrone and Wendy Hughes in chapter 3.

Michele is an artist who became ill with Hodgkin's lymphoma in 1993, and whose subsequent paintings portray a remarkable journey through the experience of illness. He was dependent on the high-tech skills and expertise of numerous health care professionals. Michele's central message to doctors and nurses is the reminder that he is first and foremost a *person* to whom something terrible has happened. He is not, as another patient he quotes puts it so well, an 'illness with a person attached'.[14]

Michele tells how the sharing of common humanity with the professionals caring for him was not only comforting, but also integral to what was good in the care he received. He is quite clear that a caring doctor is not just a nicer one, but in fact a better one. Reading Michele's piece also makes clear the value of patient narratives – as distinct from clinical histories – in enabling practitioners to understand what 'patient needs' might really mean.

Wendy Hughes is a professional writer affected by Stickler's Syndrome, an inherited disorder affecting the eyes and the joints. A selection of her work is included, along with a brief discussion of students' reactions to these pieces.

Fostering creativity

The practice of education, including medical education, is generally agreed to be pretty poorly evidenced.[15] If medical humanities is to gain acceptance as a credible academic discipline, then adopting a professional approach to evaluating these courses is desirable.[16] The creative efforts of the participants are integral to many of these courses, and these can contribute both to the formative and summative assessment of students' achievements. Scrutiny of these creative products provides one way of assessing whether educational objectives have been met. Chapter 4 describes the fostering of creativity in our own courses, and is concluded by three pieces of creative writing from students.

Conclusion

The humanities place expressing, exploring and interpreting the human condition as central to human philosophical and artistic endeavour.[17] It is the deceptively simple imperative to health care practitioners to make these pursuits integral to their daily clinical practice, which is fundamental to the humane practice of medicine. Medical humanities can facilitate access to the arts, which can provide a key to the accumulated wisdom of many lifetimes.

Notes and references

1 Cassell EJ. *The place of the humanities in medicine.* New York: The Hastings Centre, 1984.
2 The more science lays bare the complexity of what it is to be human the greater our awe at the intrinsic beauty of the human organism (see chapter 6). However doctors and healthcare legislators can lose sight of the subject at the heart of their endeavours and the results are sometimes less than beautiful (see chapter 9).
3 General Medical Council. *Tomorrow's doctors: recommendations on undergraduate medical education.* London: General Medical Council, 1993.
4 See chapter 7.
5 See reference 3.
6 Kirklin D, Meakin R, Singh S, Lloyd M. Living with and dying from cancer: a humanities special study module *J Med Ethics: Medical Humanities* 2000;**26**:51–54.

7 Macnaughton J. The humanities in medical education: context, outcomes and structures. *J Med Ethics: Medical Humanities* 2000;**26**:23–30.

8 Downie RS, Hendry RA, McNaughton RJ, *et al.* Humanising medicine: a special study module *Medical Education* 1977;**31(4)**:276–8.

9 Kirklin D, Lloyd M, Mitchell H. Special study modules in UK medical schools: a comprehensive survey of courses offered and choices made. (Paper in progress.)

10 Bristol Royal Infirmary Inquiry. *Interim report: removal and retention of human material.* May 2000.

11 Professor Robin Downie raised this issue at the Royal Society of Arts conference, 'The healing arts: the role of the humanities in medical education', by pondering the question of who might be the best teachers for such courses. Would it be doctors, literature specialists, philosophers?

12 See chapter 5.

13 Harris M. *Odd man out.* London: Pavilion Books, 1996.

14 See page 34.

15 Hutchinson L. Evaluating and researching the effectiveness of educational interventions. *BMJ* 1999;**318(7193)**:1267–9.

16 Meakin R, Kirklin D. Medical humanities: making better doctors or just happier ones? *J Med Ethics: Medical Humanities* 2000;**26**:49–50.

17 Hurwitz B. Narrative and the practice of medicine. *Lancet* 2000;**356(9247)**: 2086–9.

CHAPTER ONE

Creating space to reflect and connect

Deborah Kirklin

For many doctors not directly involved in this embryonic field, the question remains of exactly what medical humanities has to do with them, and whether it is anything more than a nice way to spend the afternoon.[1]

In this chapter I will explore two educational objectives which between them encompass much of what medical humanities purports to achieve. The first objective is to allow practitioners to reflect on their own thoughts, feelings, inclinations, practice and experience. This process of reflection offers them the opportunity to gain new insights into the strengths and weaknesses of their own practice.[2] The second objective is to allow practitioners to further appreciate the experience of illness for patients and their carers. This process is sometimes referred to as 'improving empathy'. One view of empathy as vicarious introspection comes close to describing the way in which the arts can connect doctors and patients. Both objectives require the practitioners to step outside of their professional role and to think, feel and listen person to person, and not professional to patient. I will illustrate what all of this means, in practice, by examples from my own teaching with paediatric gastroenterologists, GP registrars, clinical undergraduates and first year medical students.

A funny kind of cat

Paediatric gastroenterology might at first seem an odd place to find medical humanities. It is after all a field where scientific understanding has increased remarkably in recent years and where the tools to diagnose and treat gastrointestinal disorders in children are being developed by rigorous scientific research.[3] It is also a busy, often hectic, specialty with reflective time usually spent focusing on case presentations, audit of outcome and clinical research. One recent afternoon, instead, Professor Walker-Smith and his team at our hospital studied a piece of prose – the centre of their attention for an hour or so.

The piece, 'A funny kind of cat', is an extract from Louis de Bernieres' *Captain Corelli's mandolin*.[4] It describes how Lemoni, a little girl, calls on Dr Iannis, the island doctor, to cure a funny kind of cat with a headache. Dr Iannis finds himself led by an insistent and expectant Lemoni, on his knees through the thick undergrowth, only to find a pine marten caught on barbed wire. His instinct, to end its suffering, is over-ridden by an indignant Lemoni and he successfully nurses it back to health.

Reading through this delightful piece the group became quietly animated with many smiles and chuckles, and they had little difficulty talking about Lemoni's expectations of Dr Iannis, how he felt about children and the conflicts of interest he faced. They found Lemoni determined, confident and single-minded, expecting Dr Iannis to fulfil his role as healer without question. A negotiating dialogue rapidly replaces the doctor's initially benevolent but patronising attitude towards Lemoni as he attempts to balance his appraisal of the situation with her demands. Dr Iannis describes childhood as 'the only time in your life when madness is not only allowed but also obligatory', and acknowledges, in recognition of Lemoni's greater initial humanity when faced with the animal's suffering, that 'children see things that adults don't'.

Dr Iannis, asked to take responsibility for the funny kind of cat, faces several conflicts of interest. Instead of winning praise for a political argument he intends to put at his club, he is faced with the indignity of crawling on his hands and knees through the undergrowth. Instead of a welcome cup of coffee, trouble is in store at home because his trousers are torn and filthy. Despite all of this Dr Iannis, initially irritated and confused by Lemoni's request, finds himself satisfied and happy with the results of his labour.

Paediatric gastroenterologists get presented with all sorts of funny kinds of cat, and indeed they confided there were several on the ward that day. These doctors acknowledged their own confusion and irritation when asked to take responsibility in such cases, and the conflicts of interest inherent in medical practice were familiar to them. They also recognised that once past the confusion and irritation about what they are being asked to do, they have often found that their patients see things which they have not. Responding to the needs of these 'funny kinds of cat' can provide the sort of deep satisfaction that keeps most of us going.

All this and more came out of a discussion of this short piece of literature. Those involved gained an insight into their own practice, which they found both enjoyable and enlightening. They valued the opportunity to step back from the day-to-day pressures of their work and to think about what they do, and what it is patients hope they will do. Stepping outside their own role for an hour allowed these doctors room to begin to explore the richness as well as the frustrations of the doctor's calling.

The doer of good

Oscar Wilde's parable 'The doer of good'[5] portrays an unidentified figure who walks through a beautiful city encountering the beneficiaries of his good deeds. However, the restored functions of those he encounters are not being used as he would wish. The once blind man now uses his sight to ogle women; the man once lame now leads a wild and decadent life. Finally the Doer of Good meets a weeping man and asks him why he weeps. The answer is 'For I was dead and you made me alive. What else should I do but weep?'

I have used this piece with, amongst others, GP registrars who requested discussion of the ethical issues concerning consent. One such session took place in the week the interim Bristol report into organ retention was published.[6] Consent, duty of care and autonomy can seem rather theoretical subjects to idealistic young doctors who intend only to do good. Recent developments at Alder Hey Hospital in Liverpool and elsewhere, where childrens' organs were retained without seeking parental consent, have shown that good intentions are not enough.[7]

The first reaction among registrars accustomed to being taught about practice management, the management of chronic disease and how to pass the MRCGP, was summed up by one of them who said 'It's *so* Oscar Wilde.' Shared delight in meeting this old friend immediately took them out of role, and enabled them to respond to the piece as individuals rather than as would-be GPs. The immediate moral message was, for them, the need to remember that there is always another side to the story, and that those who ignore alternative perspectives do so at their peril. The next chord that struck was the disappointment of the benefactor with the behaviour of those he had helped. Several registrars likened it to the patient with a smoking, drinking or drug related condition who gets 'patched up' by the doctors, only to do it all over again.

Like the Doer of Good, doctors can feel let down by patients. They fail to appreciate, in both senses of the word (understand and value), the perspective of the patient. This understanding, that wishing to do good isn't always the same as doing it, was then used to explore what had happened in Alder Hey. The decision to do good, that is to develop a collection of organs for educational and research purposes was, they felt, taken in good faith. However, because of the blinkered approach taken by those involved, other goods went unrecognised. Foremost amongst these was the right of parents to choose what happens to their children's bodies (in this case after autopsy). Moreover there was a failure adequately to assess the harms involved in alternative courses of action. The supposed harm inherent in seeking consent for organ storage from already distressed parents and the potential loss of organs for the collection (if consent had been refused) weighed heavily, whereas the potential for harm, now realised, of denying parents choice, was disregarded.

By ignoring the *prima facie* good inherent in respecting the right of those parents to choose, the Doers of Good became vehicles of harm. This is not a simple case of good or bad doctors, but rather a case of doctors who had lost sight of the bigger picture. The registrars studying Wilde's parable were able to understand what had gone wrong, using a non-judgmental and balanced approach.

Adding the colour

My third example describes teaching that makes the qualitative difference between stories of illness and case histories central to the learning experience. It involves a purposeful, albeit temporary, abandonment of the editing and ordering skills which medical training provides. At the end of the first clinical year, students at the Royal Free campus can choose between three arts-based special study modules.

One of these, 'The human impact of the genetics revolution' involves, in addition to art, literature, film and drama, a visit to a volunteer's home. The volunteer is either an individual or a family member of someone suffering from a genetic disorder. The student visits not as a medic but in a journalistic role, complete with tape recorder. Both student and volunteer understand this role change. The volunteer is asked to tell their story, and not to give the student an account of their medical history. They are asked to tell the story in any way they like, and to emphasise the parts of the story they wish. The students then return to the study group to retell the stories they have been told.

Students returning to the group are excited and enthusiastic as they recount 'their' tales. The accounts are chequered with personal details that serve to explain important aspects of how families deal with or don't deal with the consequences of a genetic diagnosis. Asked what makes listening to a person's story so different from taking their history, one student remarked, 'Taking a history is black and white. Listening to the patient's story adds the colour'.

Traditional medical training conveys understanding through rigorous scientific and clinical training. The power of the arts is to add the colour to that understanding. The arts can provide students with the vicarious introspection that will enable them better to understand not only their patients but also themselves.

Even within this deliberately patient-centred approach to defining the boundaries of patients' stories, medical editing can occur. This was revealed by analysis of the differences between the stories told by the patients and those relayed by the students to the group. In one case, for example, when asked by a student about the worst effect of her child's genetic illness, a mother answered 'sleep deprivation'. This key fact was edited out, however, when the student recounted the mother's story to the group. This act occurred subconsciously and only became apparent to the shocked student when editing in general was subsequently discussed. Further analysis made it highly likely that addressing the sleep deprivation, perhaps through provision of respite care, should be a high priority for this woman's doctor.

'The alchemist'

The alchemist by Paulo Coelho,[8] a superficially simple fable of a young boy seeking his destiny, forms a core text in a literature and medicine SSM available to Royal Free and University College first year medical students. The boy's journey takes him in search of treasure, but he discovers along the way that it is the journey itself wherein his destiny lies.

Study of this text creates a space for students to reflect, right at the beginning of their training, what it is that they see as their destiny, what kind of journey they anticipate and are prepared for, and how this journey of theirs has corollaries in everyone else's lives. Other texts are used to expand and elaborate on these ideas and in addition the students produce a piece of creative writing, in the form of a fable, inspired by something they have read or discussed on the course or elsewhere in their training.

This reflection, coming as it does at a time when they are first entering into their new roles, both as independent adults and fledgling doctors, aims to be both provocative and supportive. The question of exactly what happens when you take a bright young soul and turn him or her into a doctor is clearly important. The challenge for educators is to ensure that it is the elixir of life and the philosopher's stone that remain at the end of this process, and not just a tarry mess. Preliminary results from this course will be available shortly.[9]

Conclusion

The last few years have seen growing recognition within medical circles of the important role of the arts in health. In addition there has been increasing enthusiasm to establish a role for the arts in both undergraduate and postgraduate medical education, and in continuing professional development. At a time when the medical profession finds its culture, traditions and systems of self-regulation under increasing scrutiny, medical humanities can create a welcome and necessary space to acknowledge the conflicting demands and stresses that are part and parcel of our working lives, to examine the driving force behind our practice and to connect through our shared humanity with the individuals who entrust themselves to our care.

Notes and references

1 Meakin R, Kirklin D. Medical humanities: making better doctors or just happier ones? *J Med Ethics: Medical Humanities* 2000;**26**:49–50.
2 Bolton G. Opening the word hoard. *J Med Ethics: Medical Humanities* 2000;**26**:55–57.
3 Walker-Smith JA, Hamilton JR, Walker WA. *Practical paediatric gastroenterology* (2nd edn). Oxford: Blackwell Science, 1996.
4 de Bernieres L. *Captain Corelli's mandolin*. London: Vintage, 1998.
5 Wilde O. The doer of good. In: Small I (ed.). *Complete short fiction*. Middlesex: Penguin, 1994.
6 Bristol Royal Infirmary Inquiry. Interim report: removal and retention of human material. May 2000.
7 See chapter 9 for further details.
8 Coelho P (trans. Clarke AR). *The alchemist*. London: Harper Collins, 1995.
9 Kirklin D. *A literature and medicine special study module*. (Paper in progress.)

CHAPTER TWO

Working with the metaphor of life and death[1]

Phil Barker

I know only three things.[2] First, life is a story best understood as an evolving narrative. Moment by moment, the vagaries of experience are recorded on our own *tabula rasa*, until the book is finally closed. Second, the story of my life is illuminated, pictorially, inside my head. I hear and talk in words, but the story emerges as a lived experience: I see and feel a sense of place. And finally, it is impossible to relate any aspect of my life experience directly. I need to use a foreign word or phrase to evoke its near-inexpressibility. Life is so real I can meaningfully represent it only in metaphor.

These observations appear unexceptional. However, even where metaphor is an essential part of everyday communication, awareness of its location within discourse is not always present. Thomas Szasz once told how a medical student claimed to know what a metaphor was, but could not offer an example, saying 'my mind is a blank'. Szasz laughed, but his class of educated young people did not, and he realised that they did not really 'know' metaphor.[3] In a related vein, CS Lewis noted that:

> We must use metaphors. The feelings and the imagination need that support. The great thing is to keep the intellect free from them: to remember that they are metaphors.[4]

I am emphasising here the great paradox of communication: that we use a linguistic artifice to communicate the essence of our experience, all the time running the risk of losing this essence, as well as our audience, in the translation. The Scots, to whom metaphor is not wholly unknown, have been known to express their scorn for the too clever use of metaphor with the use of another metaphor: 'you're so sharp you'll cut yourself'.

The problems of living that we blithely call illness or health are so complex that we try to objectify them – through metaphors – perhaps as a means of containing our anxiety. The disturbance of brain chemistry, for example, that many believe lies at the root of some forms of mental illness – such as depression and schizophrenia – does not involve a 'disturbance' as we might know it in the world – a 'fracas'. Nor does this 'lie' anywhere, least of all at the base (or root) of anything. Unpicking the simple metaphors used to explain our understanding of brain chemistry also pulls the rug from under them – to employ another metaphor. The metaphorical map is not the territory. Even scientific maps are metaphorical.

This use of metaphor serves as a linguistic anchor for our confused attempts to understand a potentially ineffable phenomenon. In ordinary discourse, people talk of being 'at the end of their tether', 'unable to see the light at the end of the tunnel', 'at the end of the road', 'all washed up' – or a 'shadow of their former selves'. It is difficult to make any meaningful statement about oneself or life in general *without* recourse to metaphor.[5] As Thomas Szasz, one of the modern masters of the critical appraisal of metaphor, at least in psychiatry and psychotherapy, has noted:

> A man dies and his young son is told that he went to heaven. However, when a man dies and goes to heaven, his going is not the same sort of action as that entailed in his widow going to Italy, nor is heaven the same sort of place as Rome. A man comes home and as he walks through the front door calls to his wife, 'Honey, I am home'. (He is of course neither of these things). Like jokes, which they so closely resemble, metaphors like these cannot be explained. If one tries to do so, in the process, to use another metaphor, one succeeds only in killing them.[6]

Even where manifest physical pathology is present – as in carcinoma – the patient's metaphorical description of pain, fatigue or the perceived ebbing of the life force, do not represent a mirror image of cancerous cells. It is likely that such metaphors *are* rather than *reflect* the whole, lived experience of illness.[7]

The arts possess great potential to help us understand the difficulties of life in general, but also of complex concepts like health and illness. Great art expresses the inexpressible, yet does so indirectly. 'This is not a pipe' wrote Magritte beneath his famous painting of a large pipe. Employing his typical mischievous irony, Magritte was telling the truth and deceiving us, at one and the same time. Things just 'are'. When we re-present them, they become something else, and appearances are deceptive.

The careful and, in some cases clever, use of language can help us to get close to experiences, by approaching them indirectly. We can lose ourselves in an experience, when metaphor – whether verbal or visual – helps us 'see' something for what it really is by using a phrase or image which clearly belongs to something else, as Aristotle first pointed out. The apparent 'losing' of our selves was addressed by Robert Pirsig when he observed that if we can lose the subject–object duality that dominates much of our lives, we become at one with what we are doing.[8] This becomes a kind of 'atonement'. Through this 'at-one-ness' we reconcile our differences, even with physical aspects of our world, and can be said to 'care' about what we are doing. We can also be said to be engaging directly with reality. Alan Watts noted long ago that in the West we appear uncomfortable with anything other than a dualistic view of the everyday universe.

> On being asked how to escape from the 'heat' another master directed the questioner to the place where it is neither hot nor cold. When asked to explain himself he replied, 'In summer we sweat; in winter we shiver'. Or, as a poem puts it:
>
> > When cold, we gather round the hearth before the blazing fire;
> > When hot, we sit on a bank of the mountain stream in the bamboo grove.
>
> And from this point of view one can:
>
> > See the sun in the midst of the rain;
> > Scoop clear water from the heart of the fire.[9]

Watts was not, however, suggesting that we should 'submit' to the inevitabilities of everyday experience. Rather, he suggested:

Submission to fate implies someone who submits, someone who is the helpless puppet of circumstances, and for Zen there is no such person. The duality of subject and object, of the knower and the known, is seen to be just as relative, as mutual, as inseparable, as every other. We do not sweat *because* it is hot; the sweating is the heat. It is just as true to say that the sun is light because of the eyes as to say that the eyes see light because of the sun. The viewpoint is unfamiliar (at least until the development of quantum physics) because it is our settled convention to think that heat comes first and then, by causality, the body sweats. Thus the Zenrin Kushu says:

> Fire does not wait for the sun to be hot,
> Nor the wind for the moon, to be cool.[10]

This ancient wisdom suggests the relationship between 'things' and the concepts that we use to represent them. Thich Nhat Hanh discussed the need to bring light to the gap between things themselves and the concepts we have of them:

> Things are dynamic and alive, while our concepts are static. Look, for example at a table. We have the impression that the table itself and our concept of it are identical. In reality, what we believe to be a table is only our concept. The table itself is quite different. Some notions – wood, brown, hard, three feet high, old etc – give rise to a concept of table in us. The table itself is always more than that. For example, a nuclear physicist will tell us that the table is a multitude of atoms whose electrons are moving like a swarm of bees, and that if we could put these atoms next to each other, the mass of matter would be smaller than one finger. This *table*, in reality, is always in transformation; in time as well as in space it is made only of *non-table* elements. It depends on these elements so much that if we were to remove them from the table, there would be nothing left.[11]

I perceive a curious irony in the fact that this balance of contemporary physics and Oriental psychology is to be found in a book by a meditation master, whereas the authors of many texts on contemporary psychology, talk *as if* our human concepts – of personality disorder or schizophrenia for example – and the people to whom they are applied – patients – are one and the same 'thing'.

I vividly recall the first time I experienced the 'no-self' that Watts and Thich Nhat Hanh talk about. Almost thirty years ago, for the first time,

I prepared a corpse to be taken to the mortuary. I lost all sense of myself, and was sucked into the enormity of this engagement with a body that was alive an hour ago but was now deemed lifeless. In effect, I gave up the emotional and intellectual struggle to 'understand' what it meant for this man no longer to exist, conceptually, and as a result I experienced the 'cathedral of care'. Metaphorically the 'I' that was 'me' became lost in the necessarily careful and respectful action of dressing a body after death. When a pupil inquired of his spiritual master:

> 'We eat and dress every day, how do we escape from having to put on clothes and eat food?' Mu-Chou answered, 'We eat and dress; we dress and eat.' 'I don't understand', answered the novitiate. 'If you don't understand, put on your clothes and eat your food.'[12]

My friend, the social worker, academic, psychotherapist and Zen Buddhist monk, David Brandon, recounted a similar story, bred of the same frustrated searching. He noted that:

> Shamanic practice turns its back on Homer's Calypso and the struggle to be superman or woman. Instead it takes a paradoxical journey, in arriving back at the same place. My abbot answered my question on the day of ordination: 'What does it mean to be a monk?' 'Tomorrow morning, a Zen monk will wake up in your bed and go get some breakfast.' I could have killed him but it took me years to appreciate his response.[13]

The Irish poet and mystic, WB Yeats, appeared to have wrestled with similar questions and, ultimately, came to *know* a similar wisdom:

> Labour is blossoming or dancing where
> The body is not bruised to pleasure soul,
> Nor beauty born out of its own despair,
> Nor blear-eyed wisdom out of midnight oil.
> O chestnut tree, great rooted blossomer,
> Are you the leaf, the blossom or the bole?
> O body swayed to music, O brightening glance
> How can we know the dancer from the dance?[14]

Intuitively, perhaps, as I dressed that man for his last corporeal journey, I discovered the world of experience that Thich Nhat Hanh discussed – a world in which 'things' are dynamic and alive, and even the dead are dynamically alive to us, should we allow them to be.

By talking with people about death – especially death by suicide – I have learned that not everyone submits so readily to the simulated lessons offered by Dr Death. Although Plato despaired of poetry, experience of people in various states of ill health, especially those near death, leads me to conclude that the poet, the novelist and the artist can grasp the nuances of the inexpressible, making it not only real, but meaningful. However, the closest artists have often got to medicine has been as mere illustrators of the hardware of life. We can all feel the pain and distress of patients – often our problem is to contain that emotional knowledge. Where do we put it? The metaphorical wisdom of art and literature allows us to grow a compassion for our fellow women and men, by experiencing something of the inexpressibility of their experience, without risking our emotional selves in the process.

Health care today is being rapidly overtaken by a different kind of metaphorical language that is characterised by ugliness and its capacity to obscure meaning. Were he still with us, Orwell might include Healthspeak in the same class as Newspeak. This is especially true of mental health where, in addition to the gratuitous creation of disorders within, for example, the *Diagnostic and statistical manual of mental disorders* (DSM IV), we introduce into clinical parlance politically loaded terms such as 'seriously mentally ill', implying that there might be some people whose mental illness is a trivial affair. The language of clinical medicine, like that of politics, has always aimed to put distance between us – who assume ourselves to be sane and 'normal' – and the 'objects' of our clinical attention, concern and, oftentimes, pity. One does not need to be a Zen master, or a quantum physicist, to realise that such a distinction is illusory. It is a result of self-deceit.

The core business of psychiatry is but one form of organised response to people in great human distress. Recently, in an attempt to refocus on the human issues in mental health, I asked a group of people from around the world who had experience of psychosis to describe their descent into, and journey beyond, madness.[15,16]

In *From the ashes of experience* Cathy Conroy reflected on her many years of struggle with mania and deep alienating depression, and concluded her tale with a call for an ecological vision of social and individual human development. She wrote:

> I want to see such a vision reflected in the statutory mental health services – individual reflection about who and what people are in their lives.[17]

However, professionals often find it difficult to face their own reflections when they find them in the faces of their patients. Cathy added that:

> When there is an opportunity for modelling new possibilities, for different illuminated paths, paths with heart, true exploration of our predicament can take place.[18]

The 'pathway' Cathy alludes to here is quite a different metaphor from our contemporary notion of 'clinical pathways'. Clinical pathways have little interest in who or what people are in their lives, but merely develop a string of concepts that aim to manage another concept – the illnesses that are assumed to afflict people. Cathy recognises the danger that we might (metaphorically) lose sight of the path that has become so important to her, and calls on us to use our intuitive powers to grasp something of the awful darkness of madness, believing that intuition might afford us insights that:

> ...spring from anguish, wounding, stigma, alienation in single rooms, labels, suffering, altered consciousness, desolation and betrayals.[19]

Even a tiny insight into such anguish and betrayal might, in my view, be worth mountains of what we now – ubiquitously – call 'evidence'. However, such intuitive evidence – especially when generated by people described as the 'seriously mentally ill' – is often deemed to be inferior, when it is considered at all.

Another writer in the same book, Simon Champ, struggled with what is described as paranoid schizophrenia for twenty-three years. That he is a warm, engaging, witty and self-effacing man is testimony not only to the success of the struggles of his human heart, but also evidence of how little we understand the phenomena we label 'paranoid schizophrenia'. We can tell Simon nothing about his experience, but there is much that he can teach us. Simon noted that having begun to come to terms with the sense of bereavement felt over the many years lost to his illness, he began to see clearly the difficult path he had followed, and gained a glimpse of the new horizons ahead.

> In some ways it feels as if I've come home to myself, a self changed, a self I last felt at seventeen, and yet now I'm near forty. All those years of experiences separate me from the teenager I was, but somewhere inside I'm complete again, as I used to be then. In between, despite having schizophrenia, I've lived a full life. So what was missing? What has returned? What is that quality of being, so hard to define, that is an essential part of what I'm trying to understand, a kind of being-in-the-world – in reality?[20]

Simon Champ invites us to consider mental illness from a distinctly phenomenological perspective – asking us to empathise with the ontological problems of being in such an illness state. Such an interest in the *phenomenon* of the person in mental illness appears to weaken daily.

Many now argue that the education of all non-medical mental health professionals, but especially nurses, should incorporate more of an emphasis on neuro-anatomy and pharmacology, asserting that this will better equip nurses to explain mental illness and its treatment.[21] What is rarely addressed is the assumption that this biological and pharmacological discourse is the only one requiring development. What of our need to better understand the vexed question of personhood and the largely socially and culturally constructed meanings of health and illness? We might also ask, what of the fear of madness, not to mention the fear of deterioration and decay, that appears to lie within us all?

Some of us will have an opportunity to learn something of this through direct learning from patients – even when they are deceased. There is no substitute for such a direct education. However, we have learned about the world in a vicarious way ever since we began to tell stories round our neolithic campfires. The enduring appeal of Shakespeare is that his stories appear to hold eternal truths about the human condition. They capture many forms of psychiatric disorder. By reading these works we get a chance to get a sense of the character – as a lived experience rather than an object. Talking about his experience of playing Hamlet, the RSC actor, Mark Rylance, observed:

Perhaps that's why there are so many books written about Hamlet; yet none of them could explain what some of the lines meant. It took me eighty or ninety performances before I learned what some of them meant. There is no way you can do it with a dictionary or rational thought. It is only through play that you get there.[22]

Rylance made a critical point, not simply for those who experience what might be called mental illness, but for society as a whole. To know illness we need to get inside of the experience, we need to empathise. All health and social care professionals (not to mention other members of society) could get close to the point of Rylance's experience by immersing ourselves – as he did – in the 'role' of the patient, whatever the condition. However, this is close to psychodrama and may be too threatening for many people in health care.

Most of us learn to cope with the life and death scenario with denial, and it would be folly to ban the use of this time-honoured means of facing the distress of others. However, we might care to remember the value of reading, watching or discussing the dramatic re-enactment of a life as a fine substitute for direct experience. English literature has a hoard of works that help us to appreciate the human significance of various forms of illness. In my field of psychiatry William Styron's *Darkness visible* explores depression; Daphne Du Maurier's *Rebecca*, anxiety; Janet Frame's *Faces in the water*, psychosis; CS Lewis's *A grief observed*, bereavement; Doris Lessing's *Briefing for a descent into hell*, withdrawal; Susanna Kaysen's *Girl, interrupted*, teenage breakdown; Kafka's *Metamorphosis*, identity crisis, and Malcolm Lowry's *Under the volcano*, alcoholism. There are many more.

The great value of these books is that they are more real than reality, by virtue – paradoxically – of their distance from reality. To get this close one needs to keep one's distance, which might be a form of dramatic irony in itself. These artistic accounts occupy a different body of human understanding from that of the biological, psychological or social sciences, which employ a different kind of distance from the subject: not in any way better, just different.

In consideration of this paradox of striving towards and reaching knowledge, Rilke wrote:

Being an artist means: not numbering and counting, but ripening like a tree, which doesn't force its sap, and stands confidently in the storms of spring, not afraid that afterward summer may not come. It does come. But it comes only to those who are patient, who are there as if eternity lay before them, so unconcernedly silent and vast. I learn it every day of my life, learn it with pain I am grateful for: patience is everything.[23]

People who wish to learn the art of caring need to begin with the exercise of patience. Through patience the sap of our caring capacity rises and our capacity for healing ripens slowly within us, as Rilke suggested. It is notable that great scientists also have recognised the virtue of such patient inquiry, which yields a compassion and connection with others, if not to the whole of life. Einstein wrote:

A human being is part of the whole that we call the universe, a part limited in time and space. He experiences himself, his thoughts and feelings, as something separated from the rest – a kind of optical illusion of his consciousness. This illusion is a prison for us, restricting us to our personal desires and to affection for only the few people nearest us. Our task must be to free ourselves from this prison by widening our circle of compassion to embrace all living beings and all of nature.[24]

Einstein may have been *hinting* that we already possess all that we need to become healers. This lies within us – we do not need to go anywhere to get it. In a similar vein Wittgenstein wrote:

If the place that I want to arrive at could only be reached by a ladder, I would give up trying to arrive at it. For the place I really have to reach is where I must already be. What is reachable by a ladder doesn't interest me.[25]

Wittgenstein was adding literal force to the metaphorical view of the attainment of true wisdom expressed by Albrecht Dürer in his famous engraving *Melancholia*. The most common interpretation of Dürer's *Melancholia* is that of the defeated intellect, which seeks solace in a higher plane of existence, in the next world. On the contrary, I think that Dürer – a practised melancholic himself – saw the value of melancholia as a part of the creative process. Dürer had become fascinated with mathematics – ratio in particular – as a means of developing the perfect form of expressing reality. The central image of the winged angel of the Intellect (which is probably a self-portrait) sits staring disconsolately at a scattering of mathematical devices on the ground. These instruments have failed him, or perhaps he has simply failed to exploit their potential. Dürer appears to be saying that melancholy obliges us to seek alternative solutions to life's problems. It leads to an enhanced level of understanding on the material plane of existence – here and now – rather than on any celestial plane. The ladder, which will serve as the metaphorical steps towards enlightenment, leans – almost casually – against the wall behind the great winged figure. The enlightenment, which this representation of our intellectual selves seeks, lies just out of sight, above her head – not in the heavens as many have suggested. Four hundred years later, Wittgenstein – at the peak of his logical powers – talked like the Western incarnation of the Buddha in asserting that what he sought was already *here* and *now*. Dürer, having long since found his own incarnation of enlightenment, and logical high, would no doubt have smiled in agreement.

I have used a metaphor for chaos in the development of a model of mental health nursing practice at the University of Newcastle. The Tidal Model acknowledges the chaotic nature of human experience – predictable only in its unpredictability.[26] The metaphor emphasises the power and unpredictability of the sea, echoing the power and unpredictability of mental illness. The ebb and flow of our lives is also an echo of the delicate balance between illness and health. We breathe in and out like waves lapping at the shore. In Eastern thought the breath – the *prana* or life force – heralds life with each inhalation, and death with each exhalation. We are constantly on the tidal cusps of life and death. Life is a river of experience in which we will all, ultimately, drown. Water is a powerful metaphor for life since as a species we emerged from the sea, and all of us from the waters of our mother's womb. Water is a universal metaphor for cleansing of the spirit, and the idea of drowning is used frequently by people overwhelmed by their experiences. The power of water is also difficult to contain, and we learn how to live with its power by learning to swim or by building boats or dams.

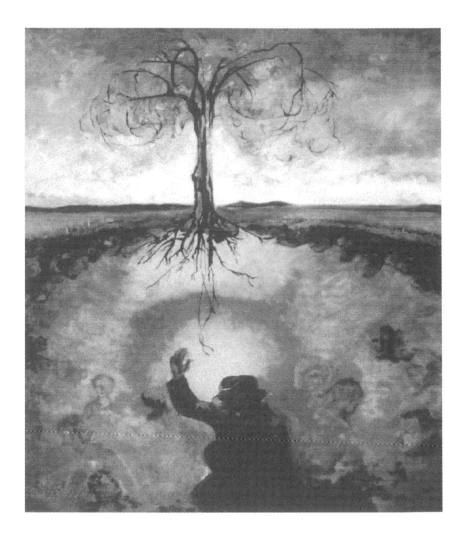

Psychiatric art   These images are a small selection from a collection of psychiatric art, the Eric Cunningham Dax Collection, in Melbourne, Australia.[27] Dr Dax has collected psychiatric art for over sixty years and I have had the privilege of viewing and discussing this remarkable collection with him several times. Dr Dax believes that, regrettably, psychiatrists, nurses and other health and social care disciplines are no longer greatly interested in the insights which might be gained from such art – insights about patients and perhaps even about themselves. Perhaps these visual metaphors take us too close to the edge of the fragile construction we call sanity.

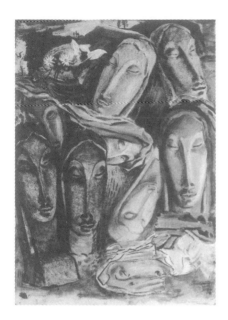

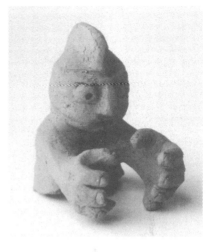

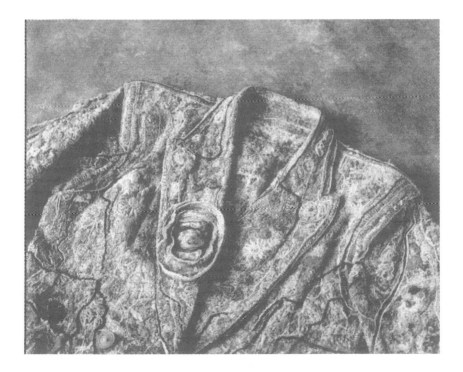

The becalming of the Ancient Mariner evokes for many people the experience of depression, especially when it is guilt-ridden. For others, psychiatric crisis is like being dashed onto the rocks, and psychiatric rescue needs to be an efficient and dramatic form of life saving. If we are to help people to understand better the weakness in their constitution (leaky boats spring to mind) or the threats that lie beneath the waterline of their lives, we need to do some repair work or deep sea diving – both metaphors for psychotherapy. At other times the health care focus is more limited in its objectives, aiming to keep people afloat – on the wider ocean of their experience.

The significance of the tidal metaphor was summed up neatly by Shakespeare, when his Julius Caesar said:

> There is a tide in the affairs of men,
> Which, taken at the flood, leads on to fortune;
> Omitted, all the voyage of their life
> Is bound in shallows and miseries.[28]

And Dickens acknowledged the tidal metaphor of life and death, when Mr Peggotty said:

> People can't die along the coast, except when the tide's pretty nigh out. They can't be born, unless its pretty nigh in – not properly born, till flood. He's a going out with the tide.[29]

These plaintive lines show Dickens's knowledge of Shakespeare, and also his intuitive empathy with the eastern notion of the *prana*.

I have regularly used the pictures from the Eric Cunningham Dax collection which accompany this chapter (see pp26–7), as well as similar pictures, in my teaching as a means of exploring our construction of the world of others – and ourselves: a world beyond words, a world of metaphorical experience that transcends description, but which is, in essence, a meta-description. As they flashed up on the screen, I have often wondered what the students thought they said about the person who made them. I have also wondered what kind of emotions they stir, metaphorically, in my student audience. What echoes might be heard within the hearts and minds, or even the souls, of individual members of the audience? What sense of meaning might be forming, silently and metaphorically, in the collective consciousness of the lecture theatre?

I am sure that one can spend a productive life in healthcare without ever considering the variegated meanings of the illness experience. If we are willing, however, to go beyond the subject – object duality that Pirsig talked about, we might foster a sense of *caring with* the person,[30] where our healing sap might begin to rise, and that might add a valuable dimension to health care. In reading books and poems, in listening to the spiritual enactments of the dramatist, in learning the discipline of studying paintings, sculpture and film we might shape a form of knowledge within us that cannot be found 'out there', but is not to be found 'inside' ourselves, either.

By augmenting our clinical education with a careful study of the various representations of the human condition found in the arts, we may learn to speak the metaphorical, symbolic language of the artist, the poet and the novelist. Such patient study may help us make a powerful connection with the human subject who is the object of our clinical attentions. Through metaphor we may gain a deeper appreciation of the human meaning of life and death. We may also learn something of the significance of our own professional lives, and our personal mortality, in the process.

Acknowledgements

The pictures in this chapter are reproduced by kind permission of the Cunningham Dax Collection of Psychiatric Art, Parkville, Victoria, Australia.

Notes and references

1 These ideas were first presented at the conference 'The healing arts: the role of the humanities in medical education', at the Royal Society of Arts, March 2000. The ideas are also addressed in a related paper: Barker P. Working with the metaphor of life and death. *J Med Ethics* 2000;**26**:97–102.
2 Given that the experience of life can only ever be personal, the personal pronoun seems appropriate.

3 Szasz TS. *Insanity: the idea and its consequences*. New York: Wiley, 1987.

4 Lewis CS. *The pilgrim's regress*. New York: Bantam, 1981.

5 Barker P. *The philosophy and practice of psychiatric nursing*. Edinburgh: Churchill Livingstone, 1999.

6 See reference 3.

7 Heidegger M. *Being and time*. London: SCM Press, 1961.

8 Pirsig R. *Zen and the art of motorcycle maintenance*. London: Corgi, 1974.

9 Watts A. *The way of Zen*. Middlesex: Penguin, 1962.

10 See reference 8.

11 Hanh TN. *Zen keys: a guide to Zen practice*. London: Corgi, 1974.

12 See reference 8.

13 Brandon D. *The Tao of survival*. Birmingham: Venture Press, 2000.

14 Yeats WB. Among school children. In: *The tower*. London: Macmillan, 1928.

15 Barker P, Campbell P, Davidson B. *From the ashes of experience: reflections on madness, recovery and growth*. London: Whurr, 1999.

16 Here I employ the term 'madness' as a metaphor for all forms of human distress, within which we might establish how to get close to such distress, whilst remaining at a distance.

17 See reference 15.

18 See reference 15.

19 See reference 15.

20 See reference 15.

21 Gournay K. New facts on schizophrenia. *Nursing Times* 1995;**91**,25:32–3.

22 Cox M (ed). Hamlet and Romeo: Mark Rylance interviewed by Rob Ferris. In: *Shakespeare comes to Broadmoor*. London: Jessica Kingsley, 1992.

23 Mitchell S (ed). *The enlightened mind*. New York: Harper Collins, 1991.

24 See reference 23.

25 See reference 23.

26 Barker P. The tidal model of mental health care: personal caring within the chaos paradigm. *Mental Health Care* 2000;**4**,2:59–63.

27 Dax EC. *The Eric Cunningham Dax collection: selected works of psychiatric art*. Melbourne: Melbourne University Press, 1998.

28 Shakespeare W. *Julius Caesar*. Middlesex: Penguin, 1967.

29 Dickens C. *David Copperfield*. Oxford: Clarendon Press, 1981.

30 Barker P, Whitehill. The craft of care: towards collaborative care in psychiatric nursing. In: Tilley S (ed.) *The mental health nurse: views from practice and education*. Oxford: Blackwell, 1997.

CHAPTER THREE

Patients' perspectives

Editor's note

In this chapter two patients-turned-teachers share their perspectives with the reader.

In 'The healing touch' Michele Petrone, a professional artist diagnosed with Hodgkin's lyphoma in 1994, powerfully argues that a humane attitude and approach from health care practitioners is not just a welcome extra but an essential ingredient in the healing process.

In 'Can't you see?' Wendy Hughes, a professional writer who suffers from Stickler's Syndrome, an inherited disorder that can cause blindness and severe arthritis, shares with the reader some of her experiences. Two poems and a piece of prose offer her perspective on the doctor's role as healer and teacher, as well as on the experience of illness for patients and their families.

Each piece contains powerful and original insights, and can arouse strong responses.[1] 'Janus' is an award-winning poem,[2] that explores the nature of the medical mask: merciful and cruel, omnipotent and vulnerable – a professional face presented to the world that conceals human failings, including the transmission of medical knowledge by the tradition of education by humiliation. The patient-witness is torn between loyalty and dismay. In 'Homecoming', the person, not the patient, is seen through a child's eyes, and in 'Where were Santa's little helpers on that memorable Christmas?'[3] humour helps make a harsh reality bearable. The tenacity and courage of both protagonists makes this a bittersweet tale.

I. The healing touch: the necessity for humanity in medicine and the humanities in medical education

Michele Angelo Petrone

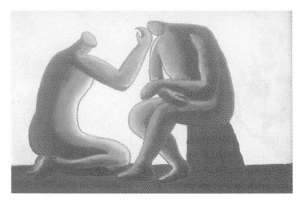

The healing touch

I need to know that this body is my body. And I need to know everything that is happening to my body. But most of all I need to know that you know that within my body there is me.[4]

Healing is brought about not just by medicine. It's not just treatment which cures you, but all that encompasses the human touch. A smile means more than an antibiotic injection, a hug means more than a platelet transfusion. The face – those of my friends, my family, my nurses and yes, even my doctors – shows sympathy, compassion and understanding. This human face contributes so much to the healing of the tortured soul.

On the 8th March 1994 a lump appeared on the left side of my neck. I had been struck down with Hodgkin's disease, which is cancer of the lymph glands. I was thirty years old. Nothing I had already been through, been taught or heard from other people prepared me for what I was about to go through in the next five years. It was more difficult and painful than I had ever imagined. But part of that pain and difficulty came out of fear and ignorance: my fear and then the fear of everybody around me. Illness and death are a part of life, yet they are very much taboo subjects in our society.

My journey has two intertwined threads, elements which mirror each other as exactly as the two chains of the double helix. One is the medical history: the physical injury, the illness, the happening, the happened, the inevitable, and the unavoidable. The parallel thread is my emotional response: the disbelief, the grief, the doubt, the flung out, the banter, the bargaining, the accepting, the clenching of teeth, the sick to the teeth, the pain, the no-gain. Why me? Why me, now?

The day after the lump appeared I went to my GP. I had never met him before. In the seven years since I had moved to my home I had not needed to see a doctor, but I knew this was important. I was living with three women, one of whom, Fiona, had been diagnosed with breast cancer two years previously. She had found the lump in her armpit, whilst changing the front door lock after a burglary. A year from now she would die in our home.

I did not tell anyone else about the lump. Perhaps I knew it might be cancer. I did not want to scare anyone else with that possibility. The culture is such that you become ill or you think you might be ill, and you go to the doctor. He told me bluntly, unashamedly, unemotionally: it might be cancer or it might be AIDS. But before they could find that out, they had to make sure it wasn't anything else. Some consolation that was. I took my blood forms, with the instructions swimming around, in my shocked state. It was clinical and straightforward, my consultation. But I was spinning, crying, screaming inside. The doctor did not know me, yet he could pronounce my death sentence. He did not prepare me, comfort me or even ask me how I felt. I did not cry in the street. I waited until I burst through my front door, whose new lock had failed to stop cancer entering once more.

The many repeated blood tests for glandular fever, and God knows what else, came back negative. In the meantime I had changed my GP, in search of someone who might include me in the consultation. I have my expertise and knowledge too, no one knows my body like I do, or how I feel. I am referred to the ENT clinic at my local hospital. I had never known where it was before, or even which one it was. Next test, cytology. Sorry, what is that? I am on this medical conveyor belt, don't know where I am going or even comprehend what it is. I trust my doctors, don't know why. But I do want to know what's happening. Can you please tell me what that means? ENT ... Ear Nose and Throat, cytology ... needle tests. Science seems to have a language all its own, which doesn't help in my emotional confusion.

Anyway they insert a needle into my lump to draw off some cells to be tested. Come back next week for the results. This time I take my closest friend. I'm called into the doctor's room. Michael, he calls me. I never knew his first name. I still call him Doctor. It's the hierarchy thing. I am vulnerable. He's not. He's big. I'm not. He's important. I'm not. That's what it feels like. My friend Bill is left outside. The door is closed behind us. The cytology tests show the type of cell found only in Hodgkin's disease. Cancer of the lymph glands. We'll have to perform a biopsy to be sure. He stares through me. No comfort. I cry alone. No word. Just silence. Alone. And my friend left outside. And as if I was left outside too. Only my lump was discussed. Tears roll down my cheek, as if invisible. And he still stares at me. We'll arrange a biopsy appointment.

Tracy's painting

Tracy attended one of the workshops I run for cancer patients, often within hospice settings. The painting she produced during that session is shown here, followed by a passage written by Tracy to explain what it means to her. I am grateful to Tracy for her permission to reproduce both.

This painting is a description of how they saw me, the me in the hospital bed. I was considered to be a patient and I was treated like a patient and this rather negated the rest of my life – the life that had been going on outside up until the moment I was admitted. It is a bleak sight; I am just a face above the sheets.

As soon as you're diagnosed the medical profession sees you as being the illness with a person attached. Actually you are an ordinary person, with something dreadful that has happened to you, absolutely dreadful. That doesn't mean that all the rest of your life isn't carrying on. Maybe you're going to have to withdraw from some of it because of the physical limits, but things like relationships will still be there. So this picture is about how you are viewed: as the illness, a cancer patient in bed, somebody who's had a colostomy. I don't blame anybody. I'm just saying that's how it feels.

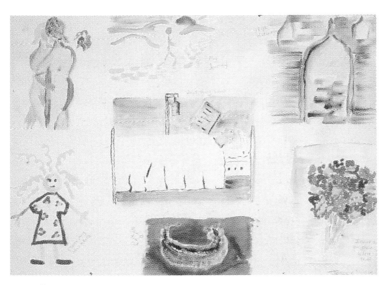

How they saw me.

I would like the medical profession to treat you as a person. You could be their sister or brother. You could be them.[5]

Tracy's painting and words encapsulate, for me, all the issues and reasons why there is this need for humanities in medical education, and humanity in medicine. Medicine is the scientific study of the human body, and treatment of the body's ills. It has always been assumed that only scientific study was necessary. The very nature of illness, of the human condition, is one of fear and apprehension. Who is not frightened of developing cancer, or even becoming mentally ill? The fear is understandable to everyone. We all recognise the emotional impact of illness, because we are all human and share those feelings of anxiety. We all feel pain, both physically and emotionally. Emotion is real.

Cancer changes everything that is familiar in our lives. We have to learn a new and exacting language, in order to express our needs, our fears and our feelings. The trauma of a life-threatening illness, and the almost unrecognisable life change, is exacerbated by our incapacity as a society to address, accept and communicate openly about the fear of our own mortality, which underlies cancer. We are all potential patients, and we will all die, yet we choose to ignore this eventuality, until it is forced upon us. Imagine then, how much harder it is, once you are affected by cancer. The world as you know it changes overnight. It is difficult to understand what is happening, let alone what you are feeling. We all dread getting cancer. Can you imagine what it might be like?

As a community, we fail to realise that one lives through illness. As an individual, the feelings that manifest themselves in each of us, are in fact a result of our being alive. The feelings of fear, pain, disbelief and anger only give more importance to the feelings of love, happiness and the value of life. How surprising it will be to some, that, through cancer, there can be very positive feeling, and a realisation that life is for living. Sometimes the possibility of dying gives permission for a way of living not previously allowed. This is not to diminish the trauma of illness, the loss, the anger and the isolation.

Freedom of expression, for all of one's feelings, is so important. A feeling also that one is not alone in feeling these emotions.

The value of painting

Communication and understanding are crucial. Through paintings and words we are able to share 'real' experiences that can inform medical practice. There are so many issues and emotions involved in the treatment and care of patients. And health professionals have feelings too. Who does not find it difficult to talk to someone who might be dying? The person assumes an aura of fragility. There is no room for mistakes. What does it feel like, to tell someone bad news? What do we do with those feelings? One must ask oneself, What does cancer mean to me?

Painting can be used as a tool of exploration. It can be enjoyable, recreational, and almost dreamlike: close your eyes and see the picture within. It can allow a freedom of expression, of emotions which may be too difficult to express in words. As the saying goes, a picture is worth a thousand words. The expression through this medium is indirect, giving an almost sideways glance into oneself, through the image. An image of the invisible, made visible through paint.

II. Can't you see?

Wendy Hughes

Janus

Observations after a failed operation for retinal detachment.

Padding removed, the surgeon explores deep within the eye.
Stony faced, he turns away and tries to mask
A tear escaping in a rare unguarded moment.
He draws up a stool and rubs the patient's shoulder.
Then, like a giant grasping at a pin, he gropes for words.

'It's difficult,' he struggles
'A complex retina, worn and fragile.'
The patient nods and understands, she needs no explanation.
The reports are clear, she knows the score.

'Another op?' she asks and then adds, 'When?'
The genius smiles,
Composure restored, the weakness breached.
'Three weeks at the earliest,' he says.

He struts into the ward
His twelve apostles billow behind.
He stops and winks,
And his patient cringes at the glint of mischief.

He reels lists of symptoms,
Surgery performed, and drugs administered.
'Gentleman, examination and diagnosis please,'
He barks, with customary arrogance.

He points to the most nervous of the bunch,
A young man steps forward, hesitates,
'You'll find the eye between the brow and cheek,' he roars.
Embarrassed, the medic bends,
Examines the offending eye
And the patient longs to help.

He explains what he can see, but as puzzled brows unite,
A diagnosis evades the group.
Then genius delivers his final humiliation,
'Ask the patient, she knows more than any one of you.'
He turns on heel and leaves,
The patient offers a smile, relaxed, relieved,
Ready to spread the word.

Homecoming

Recollections of meeting my mother arriving back
in Wales by train from London after nine months away
at Moorfield's Eye Hospital.

Hatted and gloved against the cold November winds,
We waited for the train to curl into the station.
It hissed and finally spluttered to a halt.
Through billowing smoke I watched her emerge.
I wanted to wave, to run forward and shout.
But for the moment, I was frozen
Cold words echoing through the mind.

'Things will be different now,' I was told.
'Her radiant blue eyes will never see again.
She will have changed, it may be a shock.'
I looked, she stumbled, and I tried to understand.
But to me there was no difference.
That smile, that warmth, engulfed the pain.
Mother was home; we were a family again.

Where were Santa's little helpers on that memorable Christmas?

Everyone has a memorable Christmas tucked away in their treasure chest of life.
For me it was Christmas 1958. My mother, who had been widowed two years
earlier, was determined to make this a special Christmas for me, her only child.
'It will be a Christmas we will both remember,' she said, 'one that will herald a
turning point in our lives.' It certainly turned out to be a Christmas I would never
forget, but for a very different reason to the one mother imagined.

That year had begun with a tragic event that would change both our lives
forever. On a cold February evening, as my mother was sitting making me a pair
of baby-doll pyjamas – all the rage that year – she was suddenly plunged into total

darkness. She had suffered bilateral retinal detachments, due to a genetic condition, which was not to be diagnosed until some thirty-three years later.

Mother spent most of that year in hospital, whilst I was fostered out to one family after another. It was hard for us both, but at the beginning of December she returned home. Nine operations had failed and she was told she would never see again. But as we adjusted to a new life together, Mother was determined that I would have a normal Christmas.

The week before Christmas we shopped together, and under her instructions I made coloured paper chains, and decorated the house and Christmas tree. Everything was perfect, and my mother even made a Christmas cake, which I helped to decorate with marzipan reindeers. In the excitement of preparing for the big day the sadness of the year was temporarily forgotten.

At just eight years old, I still believed in Santa. I had heard rumours of his non-existence of course, but this was still the age of innocence, and the myth was kept alive by my mother's enthusiasm and stories of conversations she had had with an army of Santa's little elf helpers. The day before Christmas Eve Mother greeted me on my return from school with the news that Annabel, one of Santa's little elves, had visited her that morning and asked if I could leave my stocking on the knob of my bedroom door and not on my bed. Apparently Santa had fallen in his Grotto and had hurt his leg, and didn't want to do too much walking around all the bedrooms, and he had requested that all good children should help him by leaving their stocking as near to the door as possible.

On Christmas Eve we prepared a plate of goodies for Santa, and a glass of milk and a few sugar lumps for his reindeer, and I went to bed wondering what Santa would bring me. I was excited, but those nagging rumours that Santa was not real kept me awake. Mother came up several times to see if I was awake and each time I spoke she seemed a little more agitated. 'He won't come if you stay awake,' she pleaded, and begged me to close my eyes. I decided not to answer Mother on her next visit to my room, and heard her heave a sigh of relief as she found her way across the landing to her room.

Minutes later she re-entered the room carrying an apple, an orange and a few nuts. The curtains had not been closed fully and with the light from the street lamp outside, I had a perfect view. Mother knew exactly where to find my stocking, and gently placed an apple above the top of the stocking. It slipped neatly between stocking and door, and rolled round and round the polished floor for what seemed like an age before hitting the wardrobe in the corner of the room. Mother stood still then tried to place the orange in the stocking, but that too slipped to the floor. Then I heard the nuts plop one by one to the floor and roll until they hit the skirting board at the far end of the room.

By now I wanted to jump out of bed, tell mother I knew there was no Santa and help her find the items, but I was supposed to be asleep! Mother, on all fours, fumbled on the floor, but could not find the objects. Undaunted, she left the room and returned with a fresh supply, a new penny and some chocolate money. Eventually the stocking was filled.

A few minutes later Mother returned with an armful of neatly packed gifts, and slowly carried them to the foot of the bed. One of the walnuts was resting in her path, and as she placed her foot on it, she began to rock backwards and forwards. As she desperately tried to keep her balance, I froze in horror. Should I get up and help, or stay silent? Whilst I agonised I watched as the top parcel began to slide and slowly slip to the floor. Mother turned her sightless eyes towards me, and listened. Then each parcel glided to the floor until Mother was left holding just one parcel. She released one hand from the remaining parcel and held the foot of the bed with the other, before sliding to the floor. I wanted to get up and comfort her, then I heard her laugh, a tearful laugh at first, which quickly erupted into an uncontrollable chuckle. She put her hand to her mouth and tried to stifle the sounds. Finally she regained her composure, and on all fours began gathering up the presents, which she placed at the foot of the bed.

I said nothing on Christmas morning about the event, and Mother seemed genuinely pleased as I told her that Santa had not forgotten me after all, and had brought me just what I wanted.

The following year she insisted that I left my stocking downstairs on the settee, making the excuse that Santa's little elf had been in touch again. Santa's leg was no better, and this year he would find it impossible to climb the stairs. Although the myth of Santa has been shattered, I still let her think that I believed.

It was many, many years later – when I had children of my own and complained how long it took them to get to sleep on Christmas Eve – that she shared this story with me. I confessed to my wakefulness and anxiety to help. She recalled her anger at not being able to fill the stocking because she wanted it be a special Christmas I would remember. Then as the parcels began to slide to the floor she saw the funny side of the situation and began to laugh. She revealed that secretly she had wished that Santa was real and that the little band of elves she had invented would come and help her find the spilled contents of the stocking. She then saw an image of herself on all fours with a little group of elves dressed in red and green weaving their way around the furniture looking for the nuts, and began to laugh. She also revealed that it was not until the summer of that year, whilst giving the bedroom a thorough cleaning, that she finally found all the nuts! It was a Christmas that I certainly will never forget!

Notes and references

1 These insights resonate with both undergraduate students and experienced practitioners in teaching settings and have stimulated exciting and impassioned debates.

2 Janus won joint second prize in a national competition organised by UK Alliance, and has been published in an anthology entitled *Happy in hospital* (Sep 2000) – an anthology of experiences by patients and those that care about them. The idea behind the competition was to publish a collection of material that could be sold in Friends of the Hospital shops, and given to patients instead of the usual flowers and chocolates. Any profits from the sale of the book will be given to a hospital charity.

3 Published in the December 2000 issue of *Best of British* magazine.

4 Petrone MA. *The emotional cancer journey.* Brighton: East Sussex Brighton & Hove Health Authority, 1997.

5 Petrone MA (ed.). *Touching the rainbow: pictures and words by people affected by cancer.* Brighton: East Sussex Brighton & Hove Health Authority, 1999.

CHAPTER FOUR

Fostering the creativity of medical students

Heather Allan, Michele Petrone, Deborah Kirklin

In this chapter we outline some of our work that fosters the creativity of medical students, and discuss why we believe this can produce benefits for both the students themselves, and for their future patients. We focus here on the creative elements of two of our courses:[1] 'Living with and dying from cancer'[2] and 'The human impact of the genetics revolution'.[3]

Creative writing

One of the creative objectives of both special study modules (SSMs) is the production of an original piece of creative writing: in the former from the perspective of someone affected (directly or indirectly) by cancer and in the latter from the perspective of someone affected (directly or indirectly) by a genetic disorder.

Later in this chapter, Ellie Cannon, a first year clinical student, writes very movingly from the perspective of a person losing their lifelong partner to cancer. This fictional account was partly inspired by what Ellie had read and heard during the course, particularly from Caroline Heler, widow of the journalist Martyn Harris. In addition Ellie drew on her personal experience: a heightened sense of the importance of one's soulmate, having got married just days before the course began. The degree to which Ellie 'got inside the head' of the dying person's lover illustrates why we so enthusiastically endorse this method of teaching; using the arts as a symbolic way of eliciting and containing personal feeling.

Following Ellie's piece, Sinead Doherty, another first year clinical student, writes from the perspective of the teenage sibling of a girl with cystic fibrosis. *Dancing Queen* is fictional, and we point this out because many of those who have read Sinead's story or who have heard her read an extract have thought it was a true account. In fact she was inspired to write *Dancing Queen* after hearing the real life story of a young woman affected by a different genetic disorder. The young woman who had agreed to meet Sinead in her home did not suffer from cystic fibrosis, but her account of how she and her family had responded to her own illness nevertheless provided Sinead with insight into the human impact of a genetic diagnosis both beyond her professional experience and beyond specific disorders.

In *Angel*, a third student, Mobasher Butt, writes a poem from a mother's perspective. The mother has a very special child – an angel. Mob wrote this piece after visiting a mother of a child with Angelman's Syndrome, a rare inherited disorder. Angelman's children are happy and playful, but never speak and have a very limited cognitive development. The poignancy of the mother's feelings for and about her child is captured in a remarkable way. There is little doubt that on this day the narrator was heard.

Creative work like Ellie's, Sinead's and Mobasher's supports the belief that humanities-based medical education can facilitate empathy or vicarious introspection. These pieces are well written and perceptive, but they are by no means unusual amongst the works produced by students on our courses.[4]

Painting

The third creative objective of the course is for the students to explore, through the hands-on use of art materials, what cancer means to them. This part of the course is run by Michele Petrone and Heather Allan. The next part of this chapter attempts to recreate for the reader the immediacy, depth of feeling, and ease of expressing emotional ambiguity these sessions can evoke.

There is an uncertainty as students arrive for the art workshop. Pencils, crayons, poster paint, large and small brushes are laid out neatly before them. 'I haven't done this since infants' school', someone says. We say only enough about what will happen for everyone to agree to attend. It's about cancer and roles, and not about being safely shut away in books or laboratories, or protected by clinical distance. What will that be like? The students don't quite know what they will have to do, if they can do it or if they'll want to. We keep it like that.

A relaxation technique takes us to a meditative state of mind. The lights are turned down low. 'Close your eyes, walk along the corridor. You come to a door. A sign on it says "Cancer". Look at the door – what's it like? What do you want to do? Do you go in? If you do, what do you see?' We hold the silence, then bring the students back to the seminar room, 'Open eyes, no talking. Reach for the paper, the brushes, the crayons. What do you see?' Ten minutes to show yourself.

The next ten minutes are full of work. Each person is absorbed in the individual interaction of mind, hand and paper. Sometimes there is a struggle. Then we have a table full of images and excited people wanting to talk. The first is Jez.

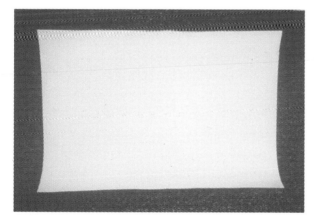

Blank thought.

Jez struggled. We have rarely seen anyone produce nothing with such intensity, working so hard at it. He is also the first to speak, and holds up a blank sheet of paper. 'This is the frustration, fear, overwhelming feeling I would have if I had to face cancer. I can't do it. This feeling came over me when I was given the paintbrush. This is not being able to do it. Not wanting to do it.' Jez very much wants to share this feeling. There is an expansion of emotional energy in the group. He's really hit on something. It can be about

45

not wanting to, being afraid, not knowing how, not being able, failing. Jez has faced, if not cancer, then a common human feeling about it, and found that he and we accept it. Jez calls his paper 'Blank Thought'. It has equal place with all the others.

Will shows us another way of not facing it, and still being part of it. His figure huddles in a container made up of the light and dark he hides his eyes from. He, himself, is made up from that light and dark. He crouches on a black ... slab? Solid ground? Grounding of knowledge and power? But that's only half the picture. The rest is left to the imagination.

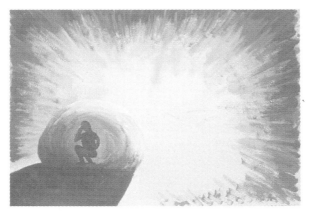

Against the light.

These students, at the beginning of their clinical training, are offered a chance to be honest about their feelings, experiencing the empowerment that can come with shared recognition, and the acceptance of their own essential humanity, including the mistakes and the frailty. Reflective work like this can allow healthcare practitioners to address the connected issues of the health of doctors themselves, as well as their own fears, anxieties and beliefs.

This idea touches on an age-old, but often unconscious dynamic in the doctor-patient relationship, which it is the task of the next artwork exercise to explore, and make available for conscious thought. It is time for more painting. With all these doubts and difficulties, what do we do? How does healing happen? How do we connect with the patient, with the predicament and within ourselves? What, we ask, is a good doctor? What does a good doctor do?

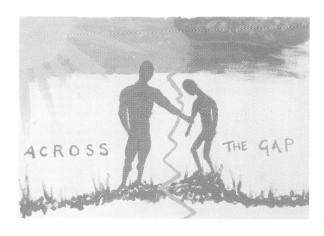

Across the gap.

This is Will's second picture. The darkness no longer engulfs the figure nor is the figure comprised of darkness, be it illness or fear or despair. There is sun and there is cloud. Two figures, in vibrant complementary colour, red and green, stand on either side of a gap that reaches from sky to ground. The arm, no longer hiding the eyes, no longer constrained by emotional denial, reaches across the gap to the arm of the other. Doctor to patient? ... Who might this 'other' be? One figure is green, the colour of natural life, renewal and healing. The other is red, the colour of danger; of feeling and of passionate energy. And each contains an image in the colour of the other: a heart and a cross. What makes this transmission possible – for the figure to stand, the arm to reach out?

To answer these questions we can use an understanding of analytical psychology, in particular, the theory of archetypes. Jung defines archetypes as 'a ... class of contents of the unconscious of an origin which cannot be ascribed to individual acquisition ... It is as if they belong to a pattern not peculiar to any particular mind or person, but rather to mankind in general.'[5] One of the integral aspects of these unconscious contents is bipolarity – as in the two figures Will has drawn. It is a picture suggestive of an archetype. Jungian analyst Adolf Guggenbuhl-Craig gives a very clear explanation of the clinical relevance of this concept, in *Power in the helping professions*.

> The healer and the patient are two aspects of the same. When a person becomes sick, the healer-patient archetype is constellated. The sick man

seeks an external healer, but at the same time the intra-psychic healer is activated ... But what about the physician? Here we encounter the archetype of the Wounded Healer.[6]

There are many expert analyses of this psychodynamic phenomenon, and its place in treatment and healing. For our purposes (and in accord with the principle of bipolarity, 'teacher/student' being another age-old concentration of psychic energy) we will let Will's picture explain.

The green figure is centred with the red heart of the other's feeling, the red figure is centred with the green cross of contradiction, crisis, and resolution: the 'wound' of the Wounded Healer. The doctor's empathy is made available to the patient by the doctor's connection with his or her own vulnerability, when this is not blocked by the denial which comes, amongst other things, from fear of being emotionally overwhelmed, or systemically unsupported. Such an attitude enables the patient to bear the 'cross', respond to the clinical understanding and intervention, with a trust which activates the unconscious healing capacity of the patient's own organism.

These are faceless figures. Their position transcends personality and reaches into the humanity in the medical dimension. 'Helplessness and weakness are the eternal experience and the eternal problem of mankind,' writes Jung. 'To this problem there is also an eternal answer, otherwise it would have been all up with humanity long ago.'[7]

The gap that Will draws splits archetypal energy, which is part of what we use to heal, into its necessary bipolarity. You need a negative and positive, a weak and a strong, a sick and a well, and a patient and a doctor to keep the show on the road. The road is the rough, natural, common ground Will paints beneath their feet. The show is our common human life.[8] Did Will come primed with a study of archetypal psychology? No; he just drew it, from, we suggest, the unconscious imprint. That's what it is. We just have to recognise, allow and value it.

Drawing conclusions

These practical art sessions allow students to acknowledge and share some of the complicated, and often ambiguous, feelings the role of healer can bring with it: a way of being connected with the other in oneself. *Night, Dancing Queen* and *Angels* (with which we conclude this chapter) show that creative writing can also offer a way of connecting with the heart and mind of the other.

Night

Ellie Cannon

You sleep now. I concentrate on your breathing. Shallow, tired breaths dragging oxygen from this lifeless grey room. Your face is calm but I know you are not at peace; your arms rest awkwardly and your body lies curled up, a position you never slept in before you became ill.

Before. Sometimes I forget about before. Our life without death. Our daily routine full of kisses, jokes, friends, wine and work. Our weekends when we escaped the city and hid by the beach or in the country. Our house, warm and comfortable, full of laughter and life. I remember the day we moved in. You were twenty-nine. Your face was tanned and glowing from our weekend in Madrid and your hair flopped over your face, the way it had done since you were fifteen. The removal vans were late and I was agitated. I paced the empty room checking my watch. They'll be here, you soothed. You had been sitting on the bare floor of our dining room reading yesterday's paper, but now you reached out for me. I sat down next to you and let your arms swathe my whole body. You were wearing your old green jumper and its warm, familiar smell mollified me. You bent down to kiss my forehead as I heard the vans rumbling down the road.

I haven't been to the house since Tuesday. As futile as it is, I stay with you like your guardian; comforting yet powerless. I breathe the air you breathe. I hear the noises you hear. I feel the twinges you feel. The ward is quiet now; nothing can interrupt us. This is our time. No drugs. No charts. No pitiful faces. We are alone and I can cup your face with my hands. You do not stir. I stroke your face, feeling every feature and memorising every detail. Your skin is still soft but you are pale. As I touch your lips you move. I watch your eyes open. You want to know the time. Late. Sleep, it's late. Go home, you look awful. You worry because I look awful. I know I do. We both smile at the irony. You know I'm going to stay. I just can't bear to leave you. You wink at me and reach out for my hand. I grasp it with both of mine. Your eyes close again and I let the tears drown me.

It is the first time I have cried in weeks. It is not bravery that stops me, it is acceptance. Acceptance. How ridiculous that we can accept it. How absurd, that there is nobody I can scream at and explain that this is a mistake. That in fact we were supposed to have another forty years together, and they got the wrong guy. Nobody will ever walk in here and say, Sorry, there was a mix-up, here's your life back. Take your wife out for dinner to celebrate. And please accept these gift vouchers with our apologies. This is what kills me: we are so bloody helpless.

When my tears finish, I leave your hand and walk to the window. You sleep again. Do you dream? I watch the night from my vantage point, my eyes following a cab on the road below. It stops and three tiny figures scramble in. I can hear distant laughter from the miniature world outside. There are no other cars to see. London is quiet. Your city sleeps with you. I think I will go home tomorrow. Just for a couple of hours. I need to have a bath, check the post, speak to your friends. There are bills to be paid. Clothes to be washed. Food to be thrown away. A life to be continued.

Life must carry on. Somebody said that to me the first time we came in here. I refused to leave you for days, terrified that if I did you would go. All those tests to be done, charts to be filled in, blood to be taken. I thought they were going to kill you. They would wheel you down to radiography and I would wait chewing my nails, praying for your safe return. Thirty minutes turned into hours. I should have gone with you, but you thought the sight of all those machines would frighten me. So I would wait. When you did come back I always wanted answers. I didn't understand how hospitals worked then – that results take days not minutes. I wanted an instant explanation. I wanted to know why my thirty-five year old husband had lost a stone over the last month. Why he was suddenly always exhausted and pale. Why he had collapsed at home on a Sunday, when we were supposed to be going out with my parents for lunch. The explanation took four days. By then I had imagined everything so I could not be shocked. I was numb. The words poisoned my ears: cancer, chemotherapy, prognosis, hair, drugs, hospital, cells, bone marrow. You asked questions. Sensible, calm questions the answers to which came and stabbed you in the back. I was silent. Gripping your hand in my vain attempt to hold onto your life. When they came in for the third time that day to take some more of your sick blood, I waited outside. The ward sister looked over to me, cautiously smiling. I did not oblige. As she approached, I stepped back. I wasn't ready for pity. This is the worst, she explained, the diagnosis. How comforting. I left my face blank. She rambled, patronised, consoled. I was an easy target. I looked young and pathetic, more like a child than a wife. She told me I should go home and relax, and that life carries on. I never did respond.

But strangely enough, it did. Here we are. Fifteen months later. Six hospital visits, two operations, two birthdays and one wedding anniversary. I sit down again, by your side. Your breathing calms me. I could listen to it all night. The blanket moves gently up and down with each breath, covering your morphine-assisted sleep. I am exhausted. I rest my head on the bed with your body. It feels warm. I start to plan tomorrow. Go home after breakfast. Bath. Bills. Phone calls. You will want visitors tomorrow. I can tell. Jenny, perhaps. I will buy you the paper and another book to read. Are you sleeping well? My mind is wandering around in the silence. I let my fingers touch you again, although this time more carefully: your sleep is precious. I stroke your shoulder gently. Do you want me to buy you chocolate tomorrow? Or maybe some fruit. You haven't eaten in days. Now the sickness has worn off, you will eat. I will get some fruit. Maybe I will ask Jenny to bring some in with her. It will make her feel useful. She can get the paper too.

Before I met Jenny I was so anxious for her to like me. I was a twenty-year-old undergraduate with no idea about the world, who had fallen in love with her older brother. She was four years younger, and still enjoying the naiveté of school and adolescence. She came to visit you for the weekend and there I was, encroaching on your time together, holding your hand when you took her to the pub under-age and staying in your bed while she slept on the floor in the lounge. I was genuinely surprised how well we got on. I thought she would hate me; I told you this when we drove back from the bus station. Your laughter filled the car, 'I ordered her not to!' She was the first person we told about the cancer. The only person we trusted with our terrible secret in those first few hours. And she is the only person who ever reacted honestly. She sat at the end of your bed and cried, swore at how unfair the whole thing was and cursed the medical profession. While other people dealt us platitudes involving the words brave and sick, Jenny spoke about cancer and chemo and even death. And the little sister I was terrified of twelve years ago became our pillar of support during a time when counsellors, specialists and even our closest friends could offer no comfort.

The night has started to fade. I think I must have slept for a while. How long, I don't know. My watch must be at home. Time has ceased to interest me. You have turned over onto your side. My neck is stiff: not a very good position to sleep in. Slowly I stand up and massage my neck. Outside the sky has brightened revealing our new day. Friday. I walk round the bed to look at your face. Still asleep. Good. My neck loosens. If Jenny comes early, I can go home, get everything done and be back by lunchtime. We don't like to leave you. It frightens me to think of you here by yourself, so Jenny is on standby at all times if I need to go anywhere. I catch sight of your watch on the bedside cabinet, half-past five. Two hours before the hospital wakes up and steals our night alone together. I rearrange the cards on the windowsill. I never read them. Their messages are trite and empty, from people who have never seen this room, who do not know the grey of the walls and the sick clinical smell.

Twelve days now, this visit. I never get used to you being here. Even when you were here for two months. Do you remember when they said you could go home? Suddenly we were acquitted from all charges and set free. You even went back to work for a while. A gesture to lead us back into normality. I stayed at home chronicling your remission, while you stepped momentarily back into the world.

You start to move and suddenly, I worry that I have woken you up again. I hold my breath to try to promote silence. But you are just turning in your sleep. Now onto your back. I breathe again. I continue making the mental shopping list I started last night. Fruit, chocolate, paper. Maybe a new book: you'll read if I buy one. Call Jenny at eight. Phone bill, electricity, car insurance. I must go to the bathroom. I walk over to the door, staring at you as I do, compelling you not to wake up. You don't. The door opens silently and I saunter down the corridor. The student nurse at the desk offers me a smile but I don't let it touch me. The ward feels cold and lifeless, and my limbs are stiff from the night's tranquillity. I can hear someone snoring and the lift outside announcing its arrival. The bathroom smells damp. I wash my face in cold water and rinse the night from my mouth. I let myself swallow the water. It tastes awful, too much fluoride. I walk back down the corridor feeling only vaguely refreshed, making a mental note to have a shower when I get home rather than a bath.

'Where were you?'

You have woken without me there and you look troubled. I approach the bed.

'In the bathroom. Are you okay?'

You nod gently, relaxing as you realise I have not gone home yet. I take your hand in mine and sit at the side of the bed.

'Is Jenny coming today?'

'Yes, I think so. I have to phone her. Do you want to see her?'

'Yeah. You shouldn't have stayed.'

You smile, trying not to sound like a scolding teacher. Your hand reaches up to my face brushing my cheek. I let you smooth over my hair.

'Did you sleep?'

'I think so. You stole the duvet again', I joke, to dissipate your worry.

'You look tired.'

'I'm fine'.

I twist my body awkwardly so my head can rest on your chest. I close my eyes and you bury your fingers in my hair. We start to breathe in unison. Your hands *comfort my head, brushing away my fear. The traffic is beginning to hum outside tapping into our peace. As I begin to relax, the nurse knocks at the door with apologies and drugs. Our night alone is over.*

Dancing Queen

Sinead Doherty

August 1996

> You can dance, you can jive,
> Having the time of your life
> See that girl, watch that scene
> Dig it – the Dancing Queen
> ABBA 1978

Shortly after my sister was born, my father and mother were informed she would never be a dancing queen. Two letters would prevent this desirable destiny, and they were attributed solely to my parents.

Certain Fadeout

Chromosome Failure

Cracked Faith

Creeping Feebleness

Certified Fatal

Cystic Fibrosis

CF

I remember nothing of this, being two years old. I am unable to recall a time when my sister, Gemma, wasn't around. Normality was Mum or Dad thumping my sister's chest, feeding her medicines or going off to visit her in hospital. I was to remain at home with one of many relatives, forbidden to visit as a potential carrier of infection.

My mother and father speak of learning of Gemma's diagnosis as an explosion of emotions. Gemma had been a smaller, more lethargic baby than myself, often wheezing or coughing, and my parents had realised something was amiss. The relief of receiving a diagnosis was immense. They would no longer be accused of 'imagining it' or 'being overcautious' by medical personnel. Proper treatment could be initiated. Gemma may finally thrive and feel better. However, the reality of CF would banish any such innocent illusions. As the doctor slowly

53

unveiled the ugly picture of cystic fibrosis, beautiful baby Gemma was transformed into a vapid victim. This was no simple childhood illness, it was a life sentence – and a death sentence. She would require constant treatment several times a day for the rest of her life. Even with such care, it was unlikely she would reach her late teens.

The agony was completed by learning the truth of how Gemma had acquired this condition – it was through genes transmitted by each of them. Frank disbelief ensued. If such facts were accurate, why did no one from either of their families suffer this affliction? How could they each carry a disease, yet be fine themselves? Why was I perfectly healthy and Gemma the opposite? That day in 1978 with Abba heading the pop charts was the beginning of a lifetime of questions, many of which would never be answered.

Recently, my mother confided that superimposed on overwhelming distress were two incredibly powerful and conflicting emotions. There was fathomless guilt at passing on such a disease; essentially she and her husband were the reason that their daughter was ill. It was undeniably their fault. But Mum was also subject to an 'unreasonably selfish' anger – feeling like a spoilt child given one gift after specifically demanding another. My mother had naturally wanted another healthy baby and had gone through nine months of hell, only to be presented with a life- long scenario of hospital visits. She would be forced to administer constant treatments to a sick child who she was guaranteed to lose. What about her own life? This was not her fault, she had not known she was a CF carrier. The anger fuelled the guilt and the guilt fuelled the anger – it was a vicious circle in danger of spiralling out of control.

My father never told us what he went through, but then he rarely discloses his feelings. When you converse with him, it is his eyes and sensitivity which betray him.

Such feelings ultimately brought my parents into closer union. It was a difficult time and they desperately needed one another, and the CF Support Society, to pull through. Many families are torn apart by such adverse news – the fact that, genetically, they have produced an illness together is understandably too much for some couples to withstand.

Gradually, my father informs me, the parameters of day to day existence changed. It was irritating and inconvenient, but bearable. Gemma required much time and energy and it was important that I did not feel relegated to the back burner. Essentially, our little family was actually drawn together by this terrible disease. This was the first of many positive points which would emerge from an initially hopeless situation.

Although I knew my sister's disease to be rare, it only dawned properly when I began school, aged four. Other children were able to run endlessly and go on any outings with their siblings. However, Gemma was not always well enough to play, and numerous trips to the beach or zoo had been cancelled as she was ill yet again. It was unfair that her CF was adversely affecting my own life (a feeling that would recur from time to time as the years progressed). My ensuing temper tantrums did little to help circumstances at home.

My parents realised the problem and ingeniously remedied the situation by gradually integrating me into Gemma's care. We would both receive prizes for behaving well on her hospital visits – prizes that most children did not deserve as they did not require such regular check-ups. I was permitted to assist in Gemma's daily physio and administer her medication – supervised by our mother at all times. It was an honour, not a chore.

Gemma and I were established playmates aged six and eight and we turned treatment into fantastic games. Medicines were magic syrup that would whisk the giver and receiver into faraway lands to have amazing adventures. We went to places that would never have been reached without the help of CF.

Madonna eloquently expressed our childish imagination at that time:

'Tropical, the island breeze
All of nature wild and free
This is where I long to be
La isla bonita.'

Gemma did miss large amounts of school due to her condition and I was often recruited to help her make up lost ground; not quite as appealing as our medicine games. She hated her inability to keep pace at sports and running. I sometimes felt depressingly helpless watching her stare glumly out the window into the busy playground, knowing I was powerless to improve her health.

Although I had temper tantrums when younger, I would realise they were nothing in comparison to the rages to which Gemma would succumb. It mystified me how she was often permitted to just scream. My dad explained the need to get it out of her system. She would wind up numb and exhausted. Usually the relatively calm few weeks following such episodes would validate my father's lenient treatment.

'Memories – good days, bad days
They'll be with me always'
ABBA

Life eventually settled into a pattern of school, home and weekends, with Gemma occasionally admitted to hospital for short periods when her health deteriorated. We both developed a love of current music, bands and having friends to visit.

Holidays were particularly special as Gemma was well enough to travel and enjoy herself. She was my sister and my best friend. We each carried on to grammar school. I noticed that she wouldn't tell all people that she was ill and I admired her for this. It would have been such an excellent excuse for submitting homework late, but she was hell-bent on appearing normal. With her sparkly personality and smile, she acquired friends easily. I watched her contend with occasionally strange reactions from friends she chose to inform. However, bad days were inevitable although the traumatic rages of younger days had somehow lessened with time.

Aged thirteen, Gemma arrived home to extremely unwelcome news. Such an event had been destined to occur, but was not expected so soon. Aaron had been a very close friend of Gemma and of our entire family. They had met whilst in hospital and stayed in contact ever since. We had been informed he was seriously ill, but had assumed he would pull through as always. It seemed impossible that a boy of sixteen would really die from CF.

Gemma was inconsolable. As I watched my sister, a well of panic I had suppressed for thirteen years erupted. I had known that CF decreased a person's life expectancy, but had refused to dwell on it. What if the same fate befell my little sister. I turned and bolted – I would never burden my family with this revelation. My sister was a ticking time bomb and nothing could slow her down.

That day, Gemma changed. A new determination appeared, apparent through her grief. She never spoke of her fear for her own life. In addition to treatment, but completely uninstructed, she started to swim. She was the slowest in the pool and it drained her. Gradually, Gem improved. By sixteen she was participating in interschool competitions, healthier than ever. She had taken health matters into her own hands – a tribute to herself and her friend. Aaron was not the only acquaintance that she would lose. Gradually and with difficulty, I realised that I could not spend the rest of my life afraid that my sister would die imminently. Such fear would force me to distance myself from her and this would be more dangerous and hurtful during her life than after her death.

'Holding on, that's what I do since I met you'
CRANBERRIES

As medicine advanced, her life expectancy would hopefully increase – perhaps gene therapy would provide the answer in time. I would make certain that the two of us would enjoy the time we had together. My parents continued to act as if they believed a cure would be discovered. This could have been interpreted as denying the inevitable, except for the fact that they tried to ensure that Gem's dreams were realised as much as possible. They did not throw treats at her or spoil her, but eventually that trip to see the pyramids in Egypt did happen, as did outings to

West End musicals and gigs in London. Living for now was as imperative as building a basis for a good future – a valuable insight that CF implanted securely in our family, and from which many others may benefit.

> *'Dancing Queen, young and sweet, only seventeen'*
>
> ABBA

Predictably, her seventeenth birthday was a massive occasion and celebration. Gem had survived to become a dancing queen against the odds. It was ironic that an Abba revival was also underway in the charts! It was noticeable that her friends purposely went outside to smoke, and that she never consumed in excess of two glasses of wine, unlike the rest of her very merry peers. Everyone was happy to accept this as part and parcel of her illness. We met her latest boyfriend who was gorgeous and keen to help with her therapy. What more could a queen desire?

I had been presented with a difficult decision a month prior to her party; should I attend a University at home, or move elsewhere? I was reluctant to leave her – the ticking time-bomb theme resurfacing – yet preferred the course offered away from our home town. I settled for a University located one hundred miles south. It was feasible for us to visit; yet we were free to lead our own separate lives.

Last week, just after turning twenty, I was tested to determine if I am a CF carrier. I have yet to receive the results. For years I have chosen not to know. Now I would prefer to discover the truth at a time when an immediate decision need not be based upon the answer, that is, my CF status is of no consequence to me, but may affect the health of my child. This will reveal whether my future Mr Perfect need also be tested. It is statistically unlikely that he will carry CF. However, should he do so, then difficult issues will need to be resolved.

Understandably, couples do refuse to produce a child who may suffer CF – they see the disease, which impairs quality of life and continually heralds an uncertain future. Yet, to have denied Gemma an existence would have been a disaster – despite cystic fibrosis she is glad that she has had a chance at life. This view is rarely expressed to my parents who refused to have a third child, fearful that he or she would be a sufferer. However, not everyone afflicted with CF is as strong as my sister. Hopefully, gene therapy may offer a new angle to such dilemmas.

Being tested has in some way inspired me to write this piece. It is not one I intend to show anyone, or read again for many years. It is a record of how I feel now, written for myself in the future. I usually avoid such activities as it makes thoughts seem final when they lie in ink on paper. It will be interesting to see how my opinions change as time, medicine and my sister's health progress.

Gem's and my own love of pop music has crept in throughout this piece. I will conclude with a quote from a new Irish band we've just discovered together. We think they will be really successful.

'We were taking it easy
Bright and breezy
We are living it up
Just fine and dandy
We are chasing the moon
Just running wild and free
We are following through
Every dream and every need
... Cos we were so young then, we are so young, so young now
And when tomorrow comes, we'll just do it all again.

THE CORRS

I hope Gem and I will be able to 'do it all again' for a long time to come.

Angels

Mobasher Butt

My new baby,
My first child,
She was beautiful,
Like a doll,
She was special.

A haughty little princess,
Insisted on being carried,
Refused to walk,
But so happy,
Never without a smile,
Constantly waving her perfect hands.

And then suddenly,
One impossibly electrifying day,
An ethereal message came from the Gods,
Transcending time and space,

My daughter was very special,
She was an angel,
My very own angel.

Maybe I too am special,
Maybe that's why I was chosen,
I had always said it,
I would be the perfect mother,
I would have the perfect child,
I have to be perfect,
My baby is an angel.

But I am not perfect,
I crave for the imperfections of normality,
I would not have chosen an angel,
I don't want an angel,
I hear your accusing cries of blasphemy,
I am drowning in guilt.

Acknowledgements

We are grateful to The Cancer Research Campaign for funding the development, delivery and evaluation of the course 'Living with and dying from cancer', and to members of the Genetic Interest Group for their help in delivering the course 'The human impact of the genetics revolution'. Our thanks go to all our fellow tutors on these courses and to our students. Working with them all has been both instructive and inspiring and this chapter is for them.

Notes and references

1 Another creative objective of both of these courses is for the students, working closely with a drama specialist, Jeanette Glasser, to use drama to portray what cancer or a genetic diagnosis can mean to those affected by it. The students work as a team to produce an original piece of drama and this is always both exciting and enjoyable for performers and audience.

2 Kirklin D, Meakin R, Singh S, Lloyd M. 'Living with and dying from cancer': a humanities special study module *Journal of Medical Humanities.* June 2000.

3 Kirklin D. The human impact of the genetics revolution. (Paper in progress.)

4 We would invite readers to visit our online anthology of student works to

experience more of the tangible benefits of arts-based medical education at
http://www.ucl.ac.uk/primcare-popsci/mhu/conference.html

5 Jung CG. *Analytical psychology: its theory and practice; the Tavistock lectures.* London: Routledge, 1968.

6 Guggenbuhl-Craig A. *Power in the helping professions.* New York: Spring, 1971.

7 Jung CG. Archetypes of the collective unconscious. In: Read H, Fordham M, Adler G, McGuire W (eds.). *The collected works of CG Jung (Vol 9, Pt 1).* New York: Bollinger Foundation, 1959.

8 The dangers of not integrating this 'humanity' are best described in *Power in the helping professions*: the doctor 'feels himself to be the strong healer; the only wounds are those of his patients, while he himself is secure against them; the poor creatures known as patients live in a world completely different from his own. He develops into a physician without wounds and can no longer constellate the healing factor in his patients ... he objectifies illness, distances himself from his own weakness, elevates himself and degrades the patient. He becomes powerful through psychological failure rather than through strength. The patient can do precisely the same thing in reverse.' (p92–5). For a brief and clear over-view of this analysis see Samuels A. *Jung and the Post-Jungians.* London: Routledge and Kegan Paul, 1985.

CHAPTER FIVE

Medical humanities for postgraduates: an integrated approach and its implications for teaching

Martyn Evans

For reasons which, I hope, will become clear, I believe I could hardly begin better than with this passage from *The Guardian* of 10th December 1998:

> Holmes and Watson went on a camping trip. After a good meal and a bottle of wine they lay down for the night and went to sleep. Some hours later, Holmes nudged his faithful friend.
>
> 'Watson, look up at the sky and tell me what you see.'
>
> 'I see millions and millions of stars', Watson replied.
>
> 'What does that tell you?' Holmes inquired.
>
> Watson pondered for a minute.
>
> 'Astronomically, it tells me that there are millions of stars and potentially millions of planets. Astrologically I observe that Saturn is in Leo. Horologically, I deduce that the time is approximately quarter past three. Theologically, I can see that God is all-powerful and that we are small and insignificant. Meteorologically, I suspect that we will have a beautiful day tomorrow. What does it tell you?'
>
> Holmes was silent for a minute, then he spoke.
>
> 'Watson, you idiot. Some bastard has stolen our tent.'

One of the faults which philosophers are most fond of pointing out in others is that of being 'in the grip of a theory' – of having one's vision wholly dominated by preconceptions about what there is to be seen at all. I am not sure whether this was more true of Holmes or Watson in the tale just told. For their immediate practical purposes, it seems that Holmes' attention to the prosaic was what was required. In the longer run, Watson's breadth of vision might have served them better, or at least more richly, if only his different perspectives – theological, horological, astronomical and so on – could have *converged* upon the more complicated phenomena of a camping holiday and how it could go well, and if only it allowed him to see the immediate difficulties as well as the deeper narrative. So – if I may pursue the homily – we need, in establishing this new field of the medical humanities, to articulate our theories but also to think and see *beyond* them. And we need to develop conceptions of medical practice and education, which are responsive to the immediate and the acute, as well as to the chronic, narrative problems of the patient. In looking at medicine from the rich variety of perspectives in the medical humanities, could we do better than both Holmes *and* Watson?

'Bolt-on' or 'integrated' humanities?

Firstly, we may ask whether the humanities are anything more than a desirable extra – in the form, perhaps, of incidental modules in ethics or literature – to be 'bolted on' to an essentially scientific conception of medical practice and education, softening and sensitising medicine's clinical application around the edges, but leaving it unchanged at the theoretical level. My own starting point is that the medical humanities should be more than this, and the teaching I will go on to describe starts from this assumption.[1]

What I shall call an *integrated* view of the medical humanities is basically the view that we need to reintegrate humanistic skills – the skills of recording and interpreting human narrative experience – into the core of medical knowledge and understanding. This involves a continual re-examination from an inter-disciplinary perspective of what medicine is, and what it is for. The teaching I will describe attempts this. The integrated view probably involves, ultimately, a reconceptualisation of what 'science' ought to mean in the medical context. This is much more ambitious, and I cannot attempt this larger question here.[2] We could say, however, that a human practice as central and important as medicine deserves no less than this.

Both a 'bolt-on' view and an integrated view of the medical humanities have strengths and weaknesses. The bolt-on or additive view has the great advantage of being easier to implement in the existing medical curriculum. Piecemeal encounters with the humanities seem quite capable of having an impact on practitioners' sensitivity when dealing with their patients, most obviously in terms of improved communications skills. The weakness of the bolt-on view is that the essential dominance of the scientific conception of the human being remains unchallenged with regard to the whole range of disease categories – including the multi-faceted, chronic conditions (think for instance of long-term angina, multiple sclerosis, organic dementia or some of the eating disorders) for which, by definition, scientific medicine currently has only partial solutions.

The integrated model of the medical humanities really does challenge this reductionist conception of the human in medicine; therefore it also (and more provocatively) claims to offer a richer approach to *diagnosis* as well as to treatment and patient management.[3] It also aims to challenge the endless subdivisions and subspecialties of clinical education and practice, which are arguably part of the problem of 'compartmentalising' the way that we think about ourselves and about each other. Moreover the integrative model seems likely to support a more far-reaching engagement between the community, artistic expression, and the promotion of personal health and well-being.

Against this, it has to be admitted that its more ambitious nature makes it more difficult to incorporate in the conventional undergraduate curriculum. The teaching that I shall describe in some detail is postgraduate, rather than undergraduate. Furthermore if the integrative model of the medical humanities were taken for a *discipline*, rather than an inter-disciplinary perspective, I would argue that it would, paradoxically, risk adding to the problem of educational specialisation and complexity. The last thing either medicine or medical education needs right now is one more subspecialty alongside all the others.

Integrated humanities

In 1995 the Centre for Philosophy and Health Care at the University of Wales in Swansea began to construct what was then an unprecedented inter-disciplinary scheme of postgraduate study, drawing together several disciplinary perspectives from the humanities, with clinical medicine as their common focus and object of enquiry.[4] A proposal for a part-time taught Master's degree was developed, following an established model of residential teaching blocks supplemented by correspondence and single-day seminars, which had served our philosophy and ethics teaching well for many years.[5] This part-time model involves a two-year taught element, successful completion of which is a prerequisite for undertaking the supervised production of a dissertation. The scheme was submitted in its present form to the University of Wales' validation procedures and, following advice from external assessors, validation was confirmed in January 1997.

A key question for the validation process was whether this was, or could be, a genuine field of academic enquiry; the external advice received by the University was favourable. The scheme was launched immediately, and the first cohort of students recruited in April 1997. In contemporary higher education modularisation is an increasingly dominant model, and the scheme was revalidated as a fully modular degree in July 1999, the general conception and content being essentially unchanged.

Obviously such an inter-disciplinary scheme cannot be either comprehensive or exhaustive in its subject coverage, so a selection of disciplinary perspectives had to be made. The five general areas we chose are philosophy, social history and politics, sociology and anthropology, literature and representational art, and theology and religious studies. One can tacitly add 'and medicine', or 'as applied to medicine', in each case. The general arrangement of the curriculum appears in Appendix A.

Owing to the disciplinary backgrounds of the principal teachers on the course,[6] philosophical reflection informs the approach to all these fields, as it forms the basis of our overall conception of the medical humanities. There is a scent of philosophical reflection when any discipline – including medicine – thinks about itself, or when a discipline thinks about how its perspective illuminates its objects. Moreover, philosophical reflection unifies, or integrates, the various disciplinary concerns that are encountered in the MA course. In effect we look, philosophically, at other disciplines *looking at medicine.*

It could be said that the humanities as a whole are concerned with recording and interpreting human experience.[7] If that be allowed, then the medical humanities are concerned with recording and interpreting the human experience of medicine. Within this general concern, when we consider social history and politics as they look at medicine we consider how medicine and health care lend themselves to being collectively organised (pondering whether it is true, as Rudolf Virchow suggested, that politics is nothing more than medicine on a grand scale[8]). When we consider sociology and anthropology, we are concerned with the idea of the *roles* – those of both the individual and the group – that are important within clinical medicine. Literature and the representational arts engage the question of how the idea of the *expressive* transcends or transforms the merely descriptive – within, and about, the experience of medicine. Social history discloses the processes within which clinical medicine has evolved and continues to evolve. Theological and religious perspectives explore the development of human narratives of suffering and salvation – ideas which, the anthropologist Byron Good suggests, have been given an intensely medical form in our present age of biological materialism.[9]

Obviously this cursory review is only a snapshot of the way we engage these disciplines; equally obviously our particular selection of disciplines themselves, and of topics and texts within those disciplines, is itself far from exhaustive. The problem of being both representative and yet at the same time highly selective in study materials confronts anyone trying to design a course like this, and so one advantage of the integrated approach is that it at least provides a unifying theme – in our case, that of philosophical reflection – to guide the choice of topics and texts, and, indeed, of humanities disciplines themselves.

The other aspect of the selection of disciplines raises the thorny problem of expertise; to deliver the course we must partly rely on visiting expert contributors from the disciplines involved. The challenge for us as philosophers is to draw out the characteristic way that medicine and health care appear from within the varying perspectives, and the expert contributors guide us in this.[10]

The main teaching format is discussion, as one might expect. This not only suits the mature age and professional nature of the students actually recruited, but it fits well with the philosophical approach – to learn to engage in philosophical reflection you simply have to have a go at it, and discussion is the best way of doing this. We explore students' individual and shared reactions to texts and presentations through discussion with them. A regular feature of the modules involves the students bringing their own choice of texts for discussion – readers who are also parents of primary school age children will be reassured to know that the current cohort (median age about forty, to judge, as it were, visually) has recently re-christened this process 'Show and tell'.

The residential format is also central to the way we teach the course. There are five short, four-day, intensive blocks where students live and work together isolated from pretty well everything except the medical humanities and sweeping views of the Bristol Channel[11] – a kind of seventy-two hour lifeboat of humanities study, from which of course it is important for them to emerge remembering that back at the surgery or the hospital it is still Monday morning and nothing has changed.

At the time of going to press we have recruited thirty-two students to the part-time course; distributed across four cohorts this number makes for highly engaged discussion, though from the viewpoint of university administration it might be regarded as somewhat labour-intensive in terms of teaching. General practitioners and midwives have been the two best-represented professional groups so far, perhaps reflecting their nature as what one might call 'narrative specialisms' (in the sense of involving a measure of continued contact with life-episodes over a period of time). Other professional backgrounds have included renal nursing, intensive care anaesthesiology, chiropractic, health care management, palliative care nursing, dentistry, and paediatric medicine. Students who apply are, of course, already interested in the subject, leaving the perennial problem of how to recruit those students who have – as one might put it – a longer road to travel. Our recruitment is initially by advertising in the specialist press and the daily broadsheets;

over the lifetime of the course this has been increasingly, and gratifyingly, supplemented by personal recommendations from students who have progressed through the course. We have been delighted to welcome students from considerable distances, some travelling from as far away as Finland and Israel. Our single full-time student to date took time out from his dental practice in Seoul, South Korea, to spend a year with us in Swansea.

It is still too early to describe formal results for the entire degree scheme, which is only now entering its fourth year. The first part-time cohort is in the final year of dissertation preparation – only the full-time student has so far graduated – and subsequent cohorts are obviously at correspondingly earlier stages of their studies. A few students have requested to convert to research degrees in identifiable medical humanities topics, and this is a resoundingly gratifying development which we have strongly encouraged where appropriate.

Challenges and opportunities

In any inter-disciplinary course the devil at one's shoulder is the risk of superficiality. The answer to this is to keep in mind what it is you are trying to achieve. In Swansea we are trying to synthesise an organic, multi-faceted understanding of medicine as a human practice. The aim, to repeat, is to facilitate not only a *sensitised* practitioner (Downie in his talk at the Royal Society of Arts called attention to the limitations on how far one can hope that study of the humanities might achieve this)[12] but one who is ready and able to reflect on the assumptions of his or her practice, and on medicine's nature, knowledge and goals.

We are therefore emphatically not trying to make mini-historians, mini-anthropologists and so forth. We consider these component disciplines to the course in terms of what *medicine* looks like to them, when they focus upon it. Even so, it is a constant challenge to us to undertake this at a meaningful and decently reflective level, and our students play an important role in keeping us attentive to this challenge, through their observations, questions and demands.

A second, connected, problem concerns assessment and examination. Again, the problem of disciplinary expertise in delivering the teaching could easily return to haunt us in this context. Therefore we set the coursework assignments with the aim of encouraging the students to consider, and to convey, how medicine appears from the standpoint of each disciplinary perspective; we also use these assignments to gauge how the multi-faceted, organic understanding of medicine is taken forward in the individual student's encounter with each new module. We have to keep the aims of the assignments, as well as the methods of assessment, under review; this is of course an inevitable feature of trying to *develop* a new, inter-disciplinary field of study – the 'benchmarks' are not given, or pre-existing; they have to emerge and evolve, and those developing the subject (including, no doubt, many readers of this volume) share in responsibility for evolving them.

One other difficulty is worth mentioning, despite bearing on only one of the five modules in the course. It is what I would describe as the problem of 'instrumentality' and it affects the study of literature and the representational arts. Unlike other disciplines – history, anthropology and so forth – which are legitimately studied for what they can *do* for us, there is a widespread and respectable view that it is improper to *use* literary and representational arts in this sense – they should be encountered solely for their own sake.[13] We have no conclusive answer to this, except to include it as an important and interesting problem worthy of the students' own attention and reflection.

It is vital in our view to be clear that the role of the humanities is to celebrate and embrace the sciences, and not to denigrate them. It is all too easy for people identified with the medical humanities to appear to be – and maybe in some cases actually to be – neglectful, scornful or hostile towards science. The last thing the medical humanities should do is to replace an uncritical 'scientism' within biomedicine with an equally pernicious anti-scientism, of the sort all too apparent in current public mistrust of medical science, and indeed of science more generally.

Having noted these challenges, I hope it will be clear that facing up to them is of course a privilege, part of the rare opportunity for students and teachers alike to share in conceiving, and pioneering in practice, a new field of study – with all the intellectual and, no doubt, professional risks which that entails.

An undergraduate innovation

In September 1999 we admitted the first cohort of undergraduate students to a new, inter-disciplinary degree, the BSc in Medical Sciences and Humanities. This scheme – developed in collaboration with the University of Wales College of Medicine – combines the approach taken to the MA just described, with study of biological sciences, combined physical sciences (physics and chemistry) and clinical sciences (including informatics). Here we have the integration of a number of science perspectives and a number of humanities and social science perspectives upon medicine, and we hope that, as it develops, this scheme will evolve and develop that more ambitious reflection on what 'science' ought to mean in the medical context. From the students' point of view, the scheme is designed to produce well-oriented and well-rounded graduate entrants to medical school, and partnership with the College of Medicine is obviously central to this.

Again, since the scheme is in only its second year, I cannot yet describe the outcomes at final examination or graduates' subsequent accomplishments; an interim report on the success of the scheme's structure should be sought from that time-honoured arbiter of the British university system, the external examiner. Suffice it for me to emphasise that the scheme is itself ambitious, from the viewpoint of students and course organisers alike (the, as it were, 'diplomatic' refinements of successfully co-ordinating the contributions of a total of ten university departments may perhaps be imagined). A schematic layout of the three year modular degree programme is given in Appendix B.

So far as I can judge, the scheme has no close precedent within our own or indeed any other established UK university. Whilst we could not, I think, be accused of academic conservatism, it is clear that the success of the degree scheme requires rigorous attention to standards and a strong resource base, as well as enthusiasm and an adventurous spirit! Intellectually, the challenge is to move beyond the mere addition of different subjects in a multi-disciplinary scheme to the *integration* of subject-based perspectives, and the mutual appreciation from within those different disciplines of the characteristic perspectives and 'objects' of the others. This is the hallmark of a genuinely *inter-disciplinary* programme of study.

The idea of a 'cultural good'

Finally, I would like to put forward a philosophical speculation, one which informs (indeed, 'drives') my conception of what it is we are trying to accomplish in these educational schemes. It seems to me that as well as being the foundation for modern health care, scientific medicine is also a special form of the way we understand ourselves, and as such constitutes what I'd like to call a 'cultural good' as well as a practical good. If culture consists, at least in part, in our attempts to give expression to how we experience our own nature and our predicament in a mysterious and sometimes hostile world, then I suggest modern scientific and technological medicine supplies us with just such a conception. It gives us the form of a distinctive kind of narrative of ourselves (even if unwittingly) in which for instance the whims of the classical deities, or the Manichean struggles of the mediaeval universe, are replaced by the probabilities of biochemical or molecular encounters; a new form of the puzzle of what 'free will' means, if it means anything at all. For all its reductionism, this narrative is a 'cultural good' insofar as it is a resource through which we can think about ourselves, our nature, and our place in the world.

But we need to transform it; to enrich its narrative, to wean ourselves away from an over-dependence on the technological salvation which bio-reductionism appears to promise us, but at the expense of a richer understanding of ourselves.[14] So our conceptions of the medical humanities might therefore also be judged by their impact on this 'cultural good' as well. I think this declares the stakes for the medical humanities to be really very high – practically, culturally, intellectually and morally – and it shows that all involved have an enormous privilege and responsibility in establishing the field and trying to take it forward.

Notes and references

1 Evans M, Greaves D. Exploring the medical humanities (Editorial). *BMJ* 1999; **319(7219)**:1216.

2 See Toulmin S. Knowledge and art in the practice of medicine: clinical judgement and historical reconstruction. In: Delkeskamp-Hayes C, Gardell Cutter AA (eds.). *Science, technology and the art of medicine.* Dordrecht: Kluwer Academic Publishers 1993, and my own interim response in Evans M. The 'medical body' as philosophy's arena. *Theoretical Medicine and Bioethics* 2000 (forthcoming).

3 Sweeney K. The consultation as Rubik's cube. In: Evans M, Finlay I (eds.). *Medical Humanities.* London: BMJ Books (forthcoming).

4 I must record here that the inspiration for and initial conception of this scheme is entirely due to Dr David Greaves, who had been gestating these ideas for several years and who continues to serve as co-director of the Master's degree course, as well as being founding co-editor of the new journal in the field, *Medical Humanities* (published by BMJ Publishing Group as, initially, special editions of the established *Journal of Medical Ethics*).

5 I refer to the taught Master's course in Philosophy and Health Care and its close successor, the Master's in Ethics of Health Care, taught in the University of Wales continuously since 1985.

6 Most of the teaching on the course is delivered by its founders, David Greaves and myself. Our academic backgrounds are in medicine and philosophy respectively, and philosophical reflection is the primary academic resource in our teaching.

7 See chapter 10.

8 Virchow R. Quoted in: Rather LJ (ed.). *Collected essays on public health and the epistemology of Rudolf Virchow.* New York: Science-History Publications, 1985.

9 Good B. *Medicine, rationality and experience.* Cambridge: Cambridge University Press, 1994.

10 We have been fortunate enough to involve a number of distinguished visiting contributors including Ms Gillie Bolton, Dr Jane Macnaughton, Dr Susan Sullivan, Dr Kenneth Boyd, Dr Mark Jackson, Professor Stephen Pattison and Dr John Saunders among others. We have also benefitted from the guidance of Professor Robin Downie and Dr Tony Hope as external examiners.

11 I should here record that from the scheme's inception until the summer of 2000 our venue was the magnificent Gregynog Hall, a mock-Tudor manor in the mid-Wales countryside, to whose warden and staff we are enduringly grateful. However, undergraduate teaching commitments have brought about a move nearer to our university campus for all our teaching from the autumn of 2000 onwards.

12 Downie R. *The undergraduate medical curriculum: being realistic about the humanities.* Talk given at the Royal Society of Arts, 30th March 2000, for the conference 'The Healing Arts: the role of the humanities in medical education'.

13 Pickering N. The use of poetry in health care ethics education. *Medical Humanities* 2000;26(1):31–36.

14 See the discussion, particularly of 'soteriology' – the understanding of suffering and salvation – in Good, reference 9, above.

Acknowledgements

I am indebted to Dr Deborah Kirklin and Dr Richard Meakin of the Medical Humanities Unit at the Royal Free Hospital for the invitation to present a version of this chapter to their conference 'The healing arts' in London, March 2000; and to Dr David Greaves of the Centre for Philosphy and Health Care, University of Wales, Swansea, both for his comments on the manuscript and for his vision in pioneering the conception of the medical humanities which is described and advocated here.

CHAPTER SIX

Caring for the whole patient: concepts of holism in orthodox and alternative medicine
A clinician's viewpoint

Michael Baum

> *Unlike science, which is concerned with the general, the repeatable elements in nature, medicine, albeit using science, is concerned with the uniqueness of individual patients. In its concern for the particular and the unique, medicine resembles the arts.*
>
> CALMAN AND DOWNIE, *LANCET* 1996[1]

The art and science of the practice of medicine have the twin objectives of improving the length and quality of life. All other outcome measures must be considered surrogates and discounted from this discussion. The objective of this chapter is to illustrate how the clinician can be an holistic practitioner contributing much to the quality of life, even amongst those patients who are predetermined to die from their condition, but also to recognise the limits of his or her own skills, at which point the role of the complementary therapist has to be defined. At the outset, for the sake of clarity of thought, I believe it is essential that we can reach some agreement about the very meaning of the words; in this case 'art', 'science', 'complementary' and 'holistic'. Having attempted to define these often ephemeral or slippery words, I will then describe in some detail the practice of a clinician as a scientist and a humanist who should recognise the limits of his or her own skills, and the point at which complementary care should be integrated.

What is art? What is science?

'Beauty is truth, truth beauty'[2]

ODE ON A GRECIAN URN, JOHN KEATS

In John Keats' famous letter to Benjamin Bailey dated 22nd November 1817, he writes 'I am certain of nothing but of the holiness of the heart's affections and the truth of imagination – what the imagination sees as beauty must be truth .... the imagination may be compared to Adam's dream – he awoke and found it truth'. In a way this could be one definition of the meaning of art in its broadest sense – the pursuit of truth about the human condition through acts of imagination such as poetry, literature, music or the visual arts. Science, the second pillar upon which Western civilisations stand, has been described by Allen Cotrell as the disciplined search for truth; in other words a search for objective realities based on sound philosophical principles which is complementary to the pursuit of 'artistic truth'.[3] It would certainly be out of place in this chapter to digress at length about the philosophy of science, but in their simplest terms the principles of modern science concern the elaboration of an hypothesis to explain observed facts, and then the testing of that hypothesis by experimentation in an attempt to falsify it.[4] The hypothesis is allowed to stand as a conditional 'truth' for as long as it can withstand robust attempts at falsification. Central to the practice of science is measurement, and if the only outcomes of importance in the practice of medicine are length of life and quality of life, then it is essential that these can be measured. The date of a patient's death is seldom a controversial issue, but the measurement of quality of life uses tools that are relatively new.[5] It is my intention to demonstrate how the practice of clinical science in the hands of a surgical oncologist can improve both length and quality of life.

What is complementary care?

There are a wide range of disciplines which are intended to complement the skills of the clinician in the totality of the care of a patient with cancer. Some are bizarre, some have little if any scientific credibility, whilst many have an important role in making the patient feel better in the corporeal domain, or live better in the spiritual domain while the clinician is attempting to cure or palliate the disease. I have no problem whatsoever with these concepts, but some practitioners of complementary medicine are intellectually dishonest and claim that they can 'heal' patients, but without providing the objective evidence required by a scientist. If challenged they will often claim to be healing the spirit, at which point the arguments get metaphysical and spiral upwards like smoke from an extinguished cigarette!

Holism as a word and a concept

The English language has a rich and beautiful vocabulary. My Oxford English Dictionary weighs several kilograms and occupies a whole shelf on my bookcase. All these wonderful words have precise meanings. It saddens me to witness how English words are being debased by a pop-culture that encourages transient values and transient meanings to our vocabulary.

Two small examples are the modern usage of the words 'clinical' and 'organic'. 'Clinical' is now used to imply a dispassionate and heartless approach to a subject where the opposite is true, in that a good clinician in medical tradition is taken to mean the wise and compassionate elder. 'Organic', a word with precise meaning in chemistry describing substances whose building blocks are hydro-carbons, is now a slippery word conveying a vague notion of that which is ecologically sound. The same worry concerns the use of the word 'holistic' when applied to the practice of medicine. The word 'holism' was coined in 1926 by Jan Smuts who used it to describe the tendency in nature to produce wholes from the ordered grouping of units. The philosopher and author Arthur Koestler developed the idea more fully in his seminal book *Janus: a summing-up*, in which he talks about self-regulating open hierarchic order (SOHO). 'Biological holones are self-regulating open systems which display both the autonomous properties of wholes and the dependent properties of parts. This dichotomy is present on every level of every type of hierarchical organisation and is referred to as the Janus Phenomenon.'[6] (Janus is the Roman god who looked in both directions at the same time). *Chambers twentieth century dictionary* defines 'holism' in a precise and economical way: 'Complete and self-contained systems from the atom and the cell by evolution to the most complex forms of life and mind'.

It can be seen that the concept of holism is complex and exquisite, and as an open system lends itself to study and experimentation. In my opinion, the hijacking of the word 'holistic' by proponents of alternative medicine is an example of debasing the currency of our language in order to prop up primitive and closed belief systems.

Holism in the organisation of organic systems

To do justice to Smuts' definition of the word holism, we have to start at the molecular level, and then from these basic building blocks attempt to reconstruct the complex organism which is the human subject living in the complex structure of a modern democratic nation state. Since Watson, Crick and Franklin described the structure and function of DNA in 1953, the development of biological holism has grown far beyond anything Smuts might have envisaged. The basic building block of life has to be a sequence of DNA, coding for a specific protein. These DNA sequences or genes are organised within chromosomes which form the human genome. The chromosomes are packed within the nucleus on an awe-inspiringly small scale. The nucleus is a holon looking inwards at the genome and outwards at the cytoplasm of the cell. The cell is a holon that looks inwards at the proteins which guarantee its structure and function contained within its plasma membrane, and at the energy transduction pathways contained within the mitochondria which produce the fuel for life. As a holon, the cell looks outwards at neighbouring cells of a self-similar type which may group together as glandular elements, but the cellular holon also enjoys cross-talk with cells of a different developmental origin communicating by touch through tight junctions, or by the exchange of chemical messages via short-lived paracrine polypeptides. These glandular elements and stromal elements group together as a functioning organ which is holistic in looking inwards at its own exquisite functional integrity, and outwards to act in concert with the other organs of the body. This concert is orchestrated at the next level in the holistic hierarchy through the neuro-endocrine/immunological control mediated via the hypothalamic pituitary axis, the thyroid gland, the adrenal gland, the endocrine glands of sexual identity, and the lympho-reticular system that can distinguish self from non-self. Even this notion of selfness is primitive compared with the next level up the hierarchy where the person exists in a conscious state somewhere within the cerebral cortex. The mind is the great unexplored frontier which will be the scientific challenge for doctors in the new millennium.

Team work and the cancer surgeon

A modern surgical oncologist is one member of a team. Any self-respecting team these days includes a clinical oncologist and a medical oncologist, diagnostic radiologist, histopathologist and clinical nurse specialist. It is my particular prejudice that the clinical nurse specialist (nurse counsellor) bridges the gap between the clinical scientist and those other disciplines that offer complementary care. My own team has immediate access to a clinical psychologist, as well as counsellors, and I have made attempts in the past to evaluate this service according to scientific principles, with the development and use of psychometric tools.[7] When I was Professor at the Royal Marsden my patients had direct access to art therapy (see below), therapeutic massage, and relaxation classes within the adjacent institute for complementary care. However, I have never recognised a role for homeopathy, special diets or any other new age 'hocus pocus' which have become more and more popular in the age of postmodern relativism. However, I do have a soft spot, or call it a personal prejudice, for art therapy, and was instrumental in developing this service at the Royal Marsden Hospital. Camilla Connell, the art therapist at this institution, published a beautiful book on the subject, *Something understood – art therapy and cancer care.*[8] I would like to quote from the preface that I was invited to write for the book, because I think it truly illustrates a recognition of the limitations of my surgical science and the importance of the integration of complementary care:

> My interest and enthusiasm [for art therapy] can be described at two levels, first there is an uncanny thematic similarity running through the works of many of these patients who face serious disease. It is as if the experience of cancer stimulates some deeply hidden communal memory to evoke the

symbolism of life and death, fear and hope. The tree, for example, is a recurring theme in these works of art, and one that can be traced back through many cultures to what may be its origin, Etz Chaim (tree of life) of the Old Testament. At the individual patient level what I found so moving is the obvious cathartic value of using art to express hidden fears, the progression of the imagery from fear to hope as a sign of recovery, and sadly in the reverse direction as a sign of deterioration. There is no doubt that art is a powerful medium for self expression for frightened patients who do not have the words or will to express themselves verbally. Good medicine is not only the practice of the science of the subject but also the practice of the humanities of the subject, and central to the humanitarian practice of medicine is the development of good communication skills. Central to the development of good communication skills is the development of empathy. Strictly speaking, empathy means trying to get inside the patient's head to feel his or her fears and pain, a task that even the most empathetic of doctors can find extremely difficult. In my experience, art therapy is the most direct line to the patient's experience of illness.

Conclusion

Complementary medicine is practised at the highest level in the hierarchy that governs the human organism. There is much research that is urgently required to investigate the psychosomatic aspects of disease and the spiritual dimension to care. Complementary therapists, therefore, should join forces with clinical scientists to explore the domain between the mind and the neuroendocrine levels of the human organism. One day evidence may show that a mind at peace with its body enhances the powers of self-healing, as a biological adjunct to the skills of a surgeon. This is a subject worthy of research, but at this point an unsubstantiated but plausible hypothesis.

Notes and references

1 Calman K, Downie R. Why arts courses for medical curricula? *Lancet* 1996;**347**:1499–1500.
2 Keats J. Ode on a Grecian urn. In: Wright D (Ed.). *The Penguin book of Romantic English verse*. Middlesex: Penguin, 1968.
3 Cotrell A. Letter to *The Times*, 1997.

4 Popper K. *The logic of scientific discovery*. London: Routledge, 1992.

5 Fallowfield L. *The quality of life: the missing measurement in health care*. London: Condor Books Souvenir Press Ltd, 1990.

6 Koestler A. *Janus: a summing up*. London: Picador, 1978.

7 Fallowfield LJ, Baum M, Maguire GP. Addressing the psychological needs of the conservatively treated breast cancer patient. *J Roy Soc Med* 1987;**80(11)**:696–700.

8 Connell C. *Something understood: art therapy in cancer care*. London: Wrexham Publications, 1998.

CHAPTER SEVEN

Art, health and well-being: why now?
The policy advisor's view

John Wyn Owen

The art of healing versus the science of healing is a very complex issue and the scene has changed quite dramatically over recent years. Sir David Weatherall, former Regius Professor of Medicine at Oxford, claims that the last ten to fifteen years have seen a change of emphasis from the whole patient and whole organs to diseases of molecules and cells, giving rise to a concern that molecular medicine is reductionist and dehumanising. Scientific medicine is often said to go back to William Harvey's discovery of the circulation of the blood in the seventeenth century, but in reality science had no impact on day to day clinical practice until the microbiology of the middle of the nineteenth century.

> Only very recently has medicine become somewhat scientific, with statistics and epidemiology applied to patient management and modern high-tech medicine, which is basically applied physiology.[1]

Diseases of western society are complex interactions between many genes, the environment we have created and the complex pathology of ageing. However a reductionist approach to disease, as exemplified by the Human Genome Project, has, paradoxically, improved our understanding of the uniqueness of each human being, and this phase in the development of medical knowledge appears to be uniting medicine and biology, rather than separating them.

> We will now start putting the bits back together again, with specialists working together and using the same technology. The old skills of clinical practice, the ability to interact with people, will be as vital in the next millennium as they have been in the past.[2]

The doctors and other health professionals of the future will need to deal with issues of enormous complexity. In the next millennium, medicine and healthcare will involve a change of focus from sickness management to health promotion by increasing use of preventive measures such as screening technology, social engineering, control of disease, non-invasive technology and biotechnology.

Humanities and medicine

In March 1998 the Nuffield Trust called together a conference at Cumberland Lodge in Windsor Great Park. Its purpose was to learn about and assess current activities, perceptions, beliefs and models of effective practice in medical undergraduate education in the United Kingdom and the United States, and about the place of the arts in therapy both in the community and in the healthcare environment.

The conference considered how to promote the practical application of ethics and the humanities in medical education and community development, in order to improve public health, the care of persons of all ages and backgrounds: the promotion of better health and well-being. The conference brought together people from different backgrounds: practitioners from the arts, philosophy, theology and many of the health professions. It also heard from those who had made innovative changes in therapy and education, both in general practice and hospitals. Participants concluded that the time was ripe for making significant intersectoral advances, involving users as well as providers.

Those taking part exchanged views on how to disseminate the information about developments in community self-reliance and ensure coordination of the efforts of public authorities and voluntary organisations. Improved communication among all those who care for the ill and who support well-being and health through the provision of the arts (such as architecture, dance, drama, literature, music, painting and sculpture) was highlighted as important. The conference recognised with much concern that failures of empathy and communication between health or social work professionals and patients sometimes exist. It was agreed that the origin of these misunderstandings needs to be understood if the situation is to be improved.

The participants recognised that some improvements in professional education and in the delivery of service can be made by rearranging existing resources. Crucial to ensuring the success of any rearrangement would be the involvement of all those in society who would be likely to benefit from changed priorities and initiatives.

Windsor Declaration: the arts, health and well-being

The conference adopted the following aims:

- ▶ to use existing resources and talents to better purpose
- ▶ to develop and expand existing skills, expertise and knowledge
- ▶ to prepare a taxonomy of what has already been achieved
- ▶ to promote collaboration in the education of health professionals by the use of distance learning and information technology
- ▶ to emphasise that health professionals need to know how to deal with people sympathetically and without condescension
- ▶ to encourage the growth of projects involving various sectors of public service and voluntary efforts.

A twelve-point action plan was developed, spanning three areas for practical application – professional education, the arts in therapy and the health environment, and the arts in community development. The relevant recommendations are that:

- ▶ medical students should be given the opportunity to study the humanities during their undergraduate education to help them develop a more compassionate understanding of the individual in society, to inspire empathy with patients and colleagues, and to become more rounded people themselves
- ▶ all university medical schools should incorporate the humanities, in particular moral philosophy, theology and literature into the five-year undergraduate curriculum, perhaps enabling the doctors of the future to qualify with Bachelor of Arts degrees, and history, creative writing and painting should also be considered for inclusion in humanities courses

▶ studying a mix of arts and science subjects should be no bar to securing a place at medical schools. If doctors are to resist gathering pressures that threaten to reduce their perceived role to that of technician, they must receive a more liberal education that helps bridge the gulf between science and the arts

▶ a national database of practice and research in medical humanities should be created in order to spread awareness and knowledge of the field, and to co-ordinate activities and encourage lifelong learning as medical professionals progress through their careers

▶ a user's guide should be produced for health managers responsible for budgeting and commissioning services concerning the practice and benefits of arts in health care and in healthy living initiatives

▶ documents should be produced on the vital contribution of arts and design in hospitals, surgeries and other healthcare settings, outlining the cost-effectiveness and the potential for improving quality of life for patients, visitors, staff and the surrounding community

▶ the notion of arts as a means of self-expression, and as a catalyst for strengthening and energising communities and enhancing the psychological, physical and emotional health and well-being of the individuals who make up those communities, should be promoted.

Progress since Windsor

The Declaration of Windsor[3] has been well received. The Committee of Vice-Chancellors and Principals welcomed the initiative and referred it to their newly-established Humanities Panel. Equally warm receptions have been received from the General Medical Council and a range of health professional interests across the United Kingdom. There has been significant media coverage.

On the 6th and 7th of September 1999 the Nuffield Trust held a second conference at Cumberland Lodge, Windsor, to take stock of what had been achieved and what future action was required to move the action plan forward in a positive and coherent way.

This conference reached a number of decisions, welcomed progress that had been made and also issued a communiqué stressing that catalysts for change are needed now to make health care, the professionals who deliver it and the people who receive it, responsive to the needs and constraints of the new century. The conference recognised the need to ensure that knowledge of what has been achieved in so many different parts of the UK, Europe, the USA and Australasia is made available and accessible to all who are interested in necessary innovation and change. As an engine of change the conference warmly welcomed the proposal to set up a new collaboration centre, the Centre for the Arts and Humanities in Health and Medicine at the University of Durham. One of the benefits such an institution would bring would be access to information, the possession of which would make it unnecessary to reinvent the wheel when innovation was being planned locally, e.g. in setting up a Healthy Living Centre, or in devising a course in art, dance or music for health.

The communiqué concluded that there was now an urgent need for a programme of pure and applied research to strengthen the evidence base underpinning the 'arts for health' movement. While social scientists had demonstrated various positive correlations in this area, the underlying causal mechanisms are yet to be explored.

The communiqué also declared that:

> People's increasing expectations of the NHS cannot be met by an ever-expanding and unlimited budget. A shift to greater concern with prevention rather than treatment will add point to a greater concern with the arts and the social content of health.
>
> All those who contribute to health care must come together with a common vision and a shared understanding that partnerships in all areas of the Health Service are vital. They need greater insight into the part the arts and humanities can play in improving understanding and empathy with patients, and with those who seek to remain healthy. If all the players can unite, they will achieve a service fit for the 21st century.

Finally, the communiqué called on the Department of Health and the Department of Culture, Media and Sport to follow the lead of the French Ministry of Health and Culture to unequivocally and clearly indicate support and encouragement for closer links between their responsibilities in the interests of good health. 'Arts for health' could play a pivotal role in the development of a new vision for the NHS that is vital to sustain and reinvigorate the service.

Among the anticipated benefits are:

▶ more compassionate, intuitive doctors and other health care practitioners
▶ patient empowerment through creative expression
▶ reduced dependence on psychotropic medication such as tranquillisers and anti-depressants
▶ growing confidence and self-reliance of individuals and communities
▶ the provision of an important approach and source of support for the combat of social exclusion

Arts and health – a third way to health gain

There is now a determined aim to elevate the arts into a pivotal role across the spectrum of Britain's healthcare and public health systems to complement the scientific and technological models of diagnosis and treatment that have driven medical policies and practice for much of the nineteenth and twentieth centuries. The role of the humanities in realising potential for health and in supporting community is summed up well by Kenneth Calman.

> The concept of 'potential' for health should be more widely recognised: potential is associated with the concept of energy – the capacity to work and play; it implies an ability to transform, to change one form of energy into another; it suggests empowerment of individuals .... Health cannot be narrowly defined; it is not just the absence of sickness, nor just about living longer, but about a better quality of life. Good health is possibly the ultimate 'feel-good' factor, and should be encouraged. Improving health is as much about employment, occupation, housing, transport, the environment, education and living standards – including poverty – as it is about treatment within the health service. This is a wide canvas, and can always be refined; the process is one of continual revision and renewal, and must therefore be grounded in values which are long-lasting and durable.[4]

Notes and references

1 Philipp R, Baum M, Mawson A, Calman K. *Humanities in medicine: beyond the millennium*. London: Nuffield Trust, 2000.

2 The Nuffield Trust. The Windsor Declaration. London: Nuffield Trust, 1998.

3 See reference two.

4 Calman K. On the state of the public health. *Health Trends* 1995;**27(3)**:71–5.

CHAPTER EIGHT

Understanding misunderstanding in medical consultation

Gillie Bolton

Many [failures] could be avoided if only the lessons of experience were properly learned.
DEPARTMENT OF HEALTH[1]

'Rabbit's clever,' said Pooh thoughtfully.
'Yes,' said Piglet, 'Rabbit's clever.'
'And he has Brain.'
'Yes,' said Piglet, 'Rabbit has Brain.'
There was a long silence.
'I suppose, said Pooh, 'that that's why he never understands anything.'
AA MILNE[2]

Understanding must be at the heart of the doctor-patient relationship. If the physician can understand the needs and wants of the patient, and the patient understand the doctor's methods and intentions, then the doctor is likely to offer appropriate interventions, and the patient is more likely to respond positively and to adopt the agreed course of treatment. Hippocrates himself stressed the vital importance of this healing relationship.[3] The ability to understand, to relate to the patient's needs and wants, is not solely brain work, as Pooh so wisely pointed out. For the doctor, understanding the patient, and understanding one's own feelings, ideas, thoughts and reactions to the interaction with the patient, cannot be separated. This understanding, or empathy, cannot be taught; but it can be fostered and developed through reflective practice writing and group work.

This chapter examines reflective practice writing, allied to carefully facilitated small group work. This can foster a range of understandings in the general practice encounter, therefore increasing clinical effectiveness. As Ron Carson points out:

> The modern dissociation of sensibility, as TS Eliot called it, according to which reason and emotion are compartmentalised, does a disservice to doctors. To care for the sick in a morally responsible manner, the doctor must delve into the patient's experience, imagine the patient's future, integrate thought and feeling, and with the patient, co-author the next chapter in a life story whose story-line has been interrupted by illness or injury. For this, literary skills are needed, the skills of close reading – a feel for pathos, a discriminating ear, a discerning eye, an analogical imagination, a way with words ... Medical education must become in this way more literate, indeed, more literary.[4]

Reflective Practice Writing courses have been delivered over the past ten years in a variety of settings in the UK. These include

- a multi-disciplinary Master's degree in Medical Science module
- postgraduate medical education courses for general practitioners (GPs) carrying accreditation, including distance learning on-line
- training for GP trainers, registrars and course organisers
- nurse in-service training, and training for supervision
- special study modules on the undergraduate curriculum
- and in-service training for full practice teams, such as primary care, child health care (psychiatrists, paediatricians, etc.), and care of the elderly.[5]

Why writing?

In speaking to others we severely, and usually unconsciously, edit what we say. On emotional occasions we sometimes edit less, blurting words out and deeply regretting them afterwards. Something spoken and heard can never be taken back. In writing, the paper (or ourselves at a later stage) is the audience. A piece of paper will not criticise, be horrified, saddened or try to interrupt. There is a safety and confidence in this. Something written for oneself can be destroyed without even being reread by the writer, and therefore unheard by anyone.

Writing is a staged process involving rereading, redrafting, editing and sharing, but only when the writer is ready. These stages enable writers to reflect and consider their work before they involve another reader; the writer can therefore afford to say more to the silent page than to an interlocutor who hears their less sifted words.

Writing is also powerful, paradoxically, because the paper keeps a record; writing is concrete, stays there on the page in the same form as when it was put there, so it can be worked on the next day or year, and then extended. Unlike thinking and talking, written thoughts and ideas can be organised and clarified at a later stage.

The writer is therefore enabled to express and clarify experiences, thoughts, and ideas that are problematic, troublesome, hard to grasp, or hard to share with another. The writer is also enabled to discover and explore issues, memories, feelings and thoughts they didn't know they had.

These attributes of writing ensure that when pieces of explorative, reflective writing are used as the basis of a group discussion, then the depth and significance of the work the group undertakes can be enhanced. A group discussion, or one with a significant reader, such as a peer, tutor or supervisor, can offer clarity and startling insight. This whole creative process can be rewarding, increasing self-confidence and self-esteem.[6] It is a process of exploration, discovery and then the integration of one's understanding about patients, colleagues and the self into professional experience.

Understanding goes both ways

The patient brings to the consultation a lifetime's worth of baggage, of which the physician will probably be aware of only a fraction, or none at all if it is a new patient. The patient similarly has no idea of what the doctor brings to the interview. A willingness to accept that the interview is deeply affected by this unknown hinterland of life experience, combined with an active awareness that it *is* unknown, is one of the foundations of a healing relationship. If the patient feels the doctor accepts them as they are, they are more likely to be open and trusting. Understanding and interpreting the patient's story, and helping them to make sense of it, is at the centre of the general practitioner's role, according to Kieran Sweeney. In doing this the doctor is inevitably affected by their own personal experience and philosophy.[7]

But so many patients present in such a way as to make it very hard to accept them as they are. A fallback method for doctors dealing with this is to respond to the awkward, unattractive, inscrutable or 'heartsink' patient by being scientific, doing no more than seeking the evidence-base for treating the symptoms as presented. They do not understand what is going on for the patient, but are being *clever* like Rabbit.

As well as an awareness of the unknown history the patient brings to the encounter, it is also useful for the doctor to recognise and examine the feelings which are aroused in them by the patient. These emotions may disable them from relating to the patient; they might be frustration, anger, fear, distress, horror or sexual attraction. One doctor commented, 'When a good looking woman walks in you can feel yourself shutting down emotionally and everything becomes clinical and removed.'[8]

There is also material within the practitioner's own experience which affects their relationship with certain issues. One GP spent much reflective practice time working through his feelings about the death of his brother when they were both children. Having done so he no longer bursts into tears with the parents of a dead or dying child, and is able to cope much better with child deaths.[9]

Reflective practice writing groups

Reflective practice, based on expressive and explorative writing and carefully facilitated group work, offers a sufficiently safe environment in which to explore issues which arise in consultation, relationships with colleagues and the work/home interface, among others. It allows an 'oscillation'[10] between examination of

a) what the patient did and possibly felt and thought,
b) what this made the doctor feel and think, and
c) the ways in which the practitioner responded – whether appropriate or not, and then, of course,
d) the ways the patient then responded in turn to the doctor.

GPs in these groups share stories or poems about specific incidents in their working experience within a small, trusted, confidential group of peers. The discussions range deeply and widely around whatever issues seem to the participants to be appropriate, yet are always rooted within the area initiated by the piece of writing. These issues might relate to prescribing, to attitude, to alternative understandings of the situation, to similar occasions when the outcome was totally different, or to relationships with colleagues. Part of the exercise is to write from the point of view of the patient, relative, or another colleague such as a nurse, as well as from their own – put simply, they write in the voice of one of the other actors in the clinical drama. The participants also imaginatively examine alternative scenarios – how it might have been different had they pursued a different course of action.

This process is a moral and ethical one. As Arthur Frank pointed out, 'Writing one's story is a moral act'.[11]

The groups always choose their own themes and write their pieces accordingly (or about a different one if a pressing issue needs to be addressed). One recent group had 'understanding' and 'misunderstanding' as its themes.

A story of an understanding

Anne is a lovely woman of eighteen or so now. A clean, fresh face, long hair, a well-proportioned, model-like figure and in the seven years I have known her, a seemingly uncomplicated person with the world ahead of her. But she has a small atrial septal defect. Two years ago she was put on a list to have it repaired. Poor thing, it has been a very long wait with uncertainty about dates.

Earlier this year she came with some somatic symptoms again, and opened up about her low mood, instability and even suicidal feelings. We talked about her situation, the operation, her protective family, her understanding fiancé, the steady work and career. She didn't seem able to make the obvious connection. She started seeing our counsellor. I put her on antidepressants and she felt better. The cardiothoracic surgeon stopped them and she got worse. I began to doubt the wisdom of operating; she seemed so healthy physically but so fragile emotionally.

93

Then I spoke to the counsellor. As on many previous occasions, I felt a surge of excitement as we talked, and it became apparent that we had the same fears about Anne's vulnerability. Then the penny dropped. Anne always wore the same sort of fairly low cut dress to display her cleavage. We thought she had it on display because her fear was that the scars from her operation would never allow her to do so again. Anne finally opened up to the counsellor about her anxiety.

I felt a tremendous urge to dissuade her from surgery until this fear had been explored. Maybe sensing this, she did not attend twice and the next time I saw her she had had the operation and was pleased with the scar, having discussed her desire for a minimal one with the surgeon.

She wore the same style of dress, with a crusty red line down her middle.

The understanding was between the counsellor and myself. I could try to use some psychodynamic approach to further analyse the situation, but lack the training or expertise. However this and other realisations that come from my discussions with the counsellor touch on my sense of inadequacy. The current term is 'emotional intelligence' and I don't know how much I possess but I want more. Highly perceptive, intuitive people have played very formative roles in my life but still remain somehow mysterious and intriguing. If I lacked this intelligence would I be able to share an understanding with such able people?

I need to find a way to open up this part of me.

CLIVE

Reflections from the group

This is a story of Clive's determination to understand not only this particular case, but to increase his potential to understand in future. The group spent considerable time unpicking what clues he might have been able to follow up at an earlier stage, and also possible strategies to foster a clearer understanding. He told us how he is considering undertaking a course in cognitive behavioural therapy; and we also discussed Balint Groups, about which I will speak in a moment. We were also able to tell Clive that in our perception he certainly does have emotional intelligence.[12] Perhaps he only needs more confidence in it and in himself, and a bit more counselling-type training. The group also pointed out to Clive that he is not a counsellor, and that the practice counsellor not only brought specific skills and experience to the case, but also considerably more time. A GP must not expect too much of themselves in terms of understanding.

Jan wrote about an Asian family whose daughters suddenly, it appeared, sought social security help and were taken into care because the father was 'beating' them. The elder girl had been anorexic and a problem for some time, and Jan had been unable to help with the situation. Jan found the case bewildering as she only saw the parents in turn (and not the daughters once they left) and each presented as completely nonplussed as to why this terrible turn of events had taken place – the father particularly.

The more we discussed it the more certain we all were that it was most likely to be a case of incest. The discussion mostly focussed around the way that so often in general practice only a small part of a situation is presented to the doctor, and how difficult it is to understand the situation from these fragments. Contrariwise we talked about the difficulty of seeing both partners in a painful or abusive marriage situation. One group member reported asking one of such a couple to see her GP partner rather than herself. We also discussed the difficulty of having empathy for a patient who has clearly harmed another, and of being an advocate for them. Jan felt much clearer about the situation, but less happy about continuing to see the father.

Caroline's writing concerned a bundle of allied problems, all contributing to making her feel stressed at work. One of these was the referral of patients for hospital consultations. She had made three referrals in one day, which made her anxious, particularly since it had been pointed out to her that she had 'the highest referral rate of all the GPs in the practice'. A very fruitful discussion followed about why and when to refer. Caroline felt reassured, but also more determined to take the sabbatical she was thinking of, and about which she had also written.

There is no misunderstanding between doctor and patient, or between GP and the hospital junior doctor, in this next story. Learning from it came from a consideration of just how this understanding was achieved.

Rosie's story

December

    'So will I be allowed to die from this?'

    'Why do you ask me that?'

    'I don't want to be kept alive. I've struggled on since my wife went, and if it's a cancer which has probably already spread from somewhere else I'd rather just get on with it.'

    'It's always your choice to be treated or not; I'm here to advise you and give you information and so is the hospital. It's your life and your choice.'

    'You think it is cancer, then?'

February

    'He just got up and walked out of the clinic.'

    'Had you given him the diagnosis?'

    'Yes, but we were discussing whether to give him chemo. He just said, 'That's it then,' and left.

    'But he'd said he wouldn't want treating. Have you spoken to your consultant?'

    'He said: ring you.'

    'That's fine. I think I said in my letter he didn't think he wanted treatment. I just wanted him to know his options and, having decided, he didn't want pressurising. He'll just have gone home.'

    'You don't think he'll have done anything ... ?'

    'No, he'll just go home and get on with living until he dies. I'll give him a ring.'

    'Shall I send another appointment; try to sort it out?'

    'I'm pretty sure he wouldn't attend; I'm quite happy to look after him. He'll come in if he's got symptoms and I can always refer him back. I don't think he'll have meant to upset you. It's just that he's a straight talker and there was nothing to say. Don't worry. I'll give him a ring and I'll speak to his daughter'.

Reflection in May

    I feel the privilege of communicating, of understanding your fatalism, your wish to decide on your own going – even if not its manner or time.

The privilege, perhaps, of unspoken like-mindedness. I know if I was in your shoes I'd choose going fishing too.

ROSIE

The patient knew what he wanted and the doctor had the wisdom to know he meant it, and to support his choice. Despite his cancer he was able to get on with his life and death in dignity and peace, as he wanted. But the GP had not only to understand and support the patient, but the senior house officer (SHO) as well. It is a heartwarming story and led to much discussion about how doctors can give permission to patients to take control of their lives (and deaths). Rosie was really hearing what the patient was saying and then respecting it. She didn't feel she knew better, and was also able to encourage the SHO to realise he didn't know better either – at least not for this man.

A member of another group wrote of a similar occasion when he was himself 'only a pre-registration houseman, shit-scared and out of my depth. I thought I had found a situation in which I knew what to do, for a change. Hence my consternation at the patient's refusal to let me.' He realised that his initial writing of the account (from his own point of view) was bald – perhaps because his memory still troubled him, unlike Rosie's. So he wrote it in the voice of the patient – and then grasped the understandings he had gained from it a great deal better. He was not only given insight, but also comfort:

Mike's poem

Leeds General Infirmary, 1982

Now this body, warped and twisted,
Has nearly reached its end, and lets its blood
Flow freely into my drug-seared bowel.

And now returning to my bedside, this tall youth
Slightly flustered, pushes an ancient drip stand.
He looks like our Ellen's youngest;
Keen, eager to do his best, but fearful he won't make the grade.
Well, fearful or not, I can't let him have his way.
'You're not putting that thing in me, young man!'

So now I lie, this quiet Sunday afternoon,
Waiting for some psychiatrist,
To try my failing faculties.
The day you gave me Lord is ending,
Now let the darkness fall.

MIKE

General practice medicine is a lonely business. Doctors in the reflective practice writing groups constantly comment on how our meetings break that silence, how they bring relationships and situations out of the closet, and open them up for supportive and critical discussion.

Balint

This 'reflections in writing' process has been likened by More to the Balint method, which:

> focusses on developing physicians' greater sensitivity and competence in dealing with their own responses to the patient, what Balint referred to as 'the doctor's countertransference to his patient' ... [and] learning to re-frame the 'problem' in non-biomedical terms.'[13]

As in the reflective practice writing groups, the participants empathise with each other within the group – modelling and practising empathy. Of course Balint relies on the physicians telling, rather than writing, accounts. In my experience reading and writing these stories offers, paradoxically, not only a deep contact with the events, situations, thoughts and feelings portrayed (for both reader and writer), but also a certain distance from them. The writing becomes a 'thing' in its own right to which the group can relate – the writer is let off the hook to an extent, and can relate relatively safely to the story too, rather than to themselves. It is of course still very exposing and often close to the bone.

Enid Balint and JS Norell emphasise the physician listening to the patient, saying that 'he who asks questions will get answers – but hardly anything else'. They also speak of: '*tuning-in* to the patient, understanding her communications and responding to them so that she would feel that she was understood.'[14]

Reflective practice writing groups and Balint groups can enable doctors to understand more fully what it means to listen and tune in, by the sharing of experiences with each other. This offers a window into the practice of others, and a supportively critical eye and ear on one's own practice. More concludes her account of a Balint group of American medical residents thus:

> The reflexive interpretive skills developed through Balint work can enhance physicians' ability to 'read' the doctor–patient relationship and their own contribution to it. Through development of empathy, they deepened their understanding of the patient's narrative and a commitment to become more responsible for the part they play in the dialogue. In this way empathic knowledge can move from understanding to responsible action.[15]

An empathic relationship

Understanding is a key feature of an empathic relationship. Rosie's relationship with her patient was clearly empathic. She was doing far more than responding to what the patient wanted. She was actively listening, and hearing what he needed and wanted. She was doing more than being sympathetic, and yet was not, and would not pretend to be, knowing and feeling what the patient was feeling. No one person can do that for another as we are all inexorably stuck in our own skins, brains and emotions. This kind of pretence makes any patient or client feel their own individuality is not being respected. Empathy is an ability to relate to the affective, physical, cognitive and spiritual experience of another. The physician is emotionally as well as cognitively and spiritually involved, but their integrity is intact – they are not personally hurt by the patient, nor do they fall in love with him or her, or become personally burdened. Although they are often left tired and distressed, this should be nothing which a good bout of reflective practice or mentoring and a rest cannot ease.

The group work enabled Rosie to explore what this incident meant to her. She was able to accept the impact of her actions upon this patient and upon the SHO. The group were also able to empathise with her, and – by proxy – the patient. This in turn is likely to give them the skill and courage to be more empathic with their own patients.

A doctor can better empathise with a patient's situation when they have examined and come to some degree of understanding about their own values, feelings and relevant experiences – through a process such as reflective practice writing and group work. There is then a sense of stability in knowing who one is in the face of the battery of material and emotions the patient brings. The practitioner is enabled to think about the patient's presenting and possible hidden problems reasonably clearly, without their own feelings and memories getting in the way too much. The patient's response to the doctor – cringing, angry, appealing, flirtatious, overbearing, motherly or fatherly – can also, potentially, throw the doctor off empathic track and into automatic response.

All these factors would be called transference and counter-transference within a psychotherapeutic relationship, where they are not only recognised, but wielded as invaluable tools. Yet, as Clive pointed out in an ensuing reflective practice writing session, 'we are not trained in any therapeutic or counselling skills at all.' Discussing experiences, and different options for how to deal with them, is the work of the reflective practice writing group. It does not offer therapeutic or counselling skills but it can open up depths of understanding of both the self and others.

Physicians feel *respect* for themselves as skilled and experienced practitioners, and they *trust* the process in which they are engaged – that of doctoring. All good relationships are built on these two foundations. A good professional clinical relationship is not exactly the same as a normal, everyday 'good' one, however. It is not based on a *personal* trust and respect, but a trust and respect of the patient as they are encountered within the narrow clinical situation. The practitioner might well feel completely differently about the individual on meeting them in a non-clinical situation. The GPs in one of my other groups considered this issue with regard to drug users. They felt they could have empathy with such people, yet would be unlikely to have respect and possibly trust for many of them, as honesty and straightforwardness, as the GP would understand them, are not in such people's experience of life. I think they meant that the trust and respect in these encounters is different from that within adult non-clinical relationships such as friendship or collegiality.

The third element in normal good relationships, in addition to trust and respect, is love. Rogers chose to use the expression: 'unconditional positive regard'[16] (the ancient Greeks would have called it *agape*) when considering the therapeutic or teaching relationship. Rosie and her patient clearly felt this for each other; it is essential to an empathetic relationship. Personal feelings of distaste, sexual attraction or protectiveness are put on one side as the physician takes on the role of professional advocate for their patient. The triumvirate of trust, respect and love are firmly present in an empathic clinical relationship – but they need to be appropriately positioned.

The physician in an empathic relationship is neither distant and unemotional, nor relating personally to the patient, but *present* with the patient.[17] They are able to communicate their presence to the patient. This, in turn, gives the patient confidence to be more present with the doctor. John Berger, writing of the GP Dr Sassall, uses the expression 'recognition': 'what is required of him is that he should recognise his patient with the certainty of an ideal brother. The function of fraternity is recognition.'[18]

Coulehan has pointed out that 'empathy is an affair of the heart and imagination.'[19] He also said doctors need '*emotional resilience, a resilience that allows one to fully experience the emotional dynamics of patient care as an essential part of – rather than a detriment to – good medical practice.*'[20] The physician is involved without being personally damaged or affected by these 'full emotional dynamics'. Yet medical school tends to train people to be unemotional. One GP even refused to be involved in a research study into 'the emotional demands of general practice', stating that it was a 'waste of time because emotions are not part of a GP's professional life'.[21]

Creative writing

Jack Coulehan has written:

> My life in poetry has taught me that empathy is an affair of the heart and imagination. [We must] call [the emotions] by name rather than ignoring them completely or attempting to sanitise them. By attempting to enter my patients' stories and in essence re-imagine them through words and

symbols, I learned that compassion, courage, self-effacement, and humour set the stage for healing ... Empathy, metaphor and imagination are really at the root of the art of medicine.[22]

As Coulehan says, sympathy can be fostered, and reflective practice rendered effective, by the writing of poetry or prose. Writing such material takes the doctor into a deeply insightful relationship with the everyday concerns of their professional life. And when those written poems or stories are shared with a trusting and confidential group of peers, an informed, deeply explorative discussion can ensue.

Stress management

Suppressing or repressing emotions can lead to burnout and lowered performance.[23] Reflective practice writing groups support practitioners towards a better understanding of their own emotions, motives and thoughts. This improved understanding can give them insight into the areas of their professional life which act as stressors, and what they can do about them. It has been observed that:

> Writing is a disinhibition strategy, as it anchors people to a safe present while they re-experience a past event, providing optimum distance possibilities and hence cathartic reset.[24]

A considerable body of randomised control trial evidence demonstrates that writing has the power to decrease stress and boost the immune system.[25,26]

Discussing such writings in a confidential and trusted forum of peers can enable practitioners to learn how to prevent areas of professional life becoming so stressful they need *cathartic reset*. Here is another story from the same group of GPs:

Jane's story

'How are you?' Not upbeat, just kind. I know the answer. So he tells me the latest rundown: old problems and the new ones. I've just seen his wife, badly depressed about carrying this burden day and night. She'd told me, 'But it's always the same.' So again we pick up on his most pressing

difficulties. I feel myself spiral down, revisiting the painful inadequacy and guilt, the fleeting wish that he wouldn't keep seeing me month by month.

I open my mouth and groan, with no preparation, no censoring. I blurt out: 'Oh Gordon, I feel so awful, I've been off for five months, I come back and you're a bit worse, Brenda's much worse and I've still got nothing to offer. I'm so sorry.' I look at the desk.

He squeezed my arm so caringly. He searched out my eyes: 'Don't worry,' he said kindly, not flattened or dispirited. 'I know how it is. It's the same at hospital. I know you can't do anything for me.' We looked at each other. 'Thank you,' I said, 'that's lovely of you to say.'

We finished our consultation. He booked his next appointment as I called the next patient in.

JANE

Now that's empathy. I think the relationship was probably already empathic before this incident, but it was Jane, the GP, who took the lead in deepening that understanding (whereas in Rosie's story it was the patient). You can imagine the kind of discussion in the group which followed Jane's story. 'How much is it reasonable for the doctor to share their feelings with the patient?' 'Might it not just have been terribly damaging what she did?' In this case it wasn't. Jane clearly trusted not only her general practice skill and experience, but also her empathic feeling for this particular patient. As with Rosie's patient, plain speaking was what he wanted. But here part of Jane's message was 'I don't know what to do'. As John Horder has pointed out: 'To say *I don't know* is essential in medicine.'[27] In this case, Jane's open acceptance of her inability to come up with answers deepened the empathic understanding between her and her patient.

The doctors in the group were able to learn from the experiences recounted in these stories, try them out in discussion against cases of their own, and hope to be courageous enough to deepen empathic and understanding relationships in these kinds of ways with patients in the future.

The practitioner cannot expect to change or improve the attitude of the patient.

One GP confessed on a Friday evening that she was simply too exhausted to relate to the complex issue with which a patient presented, and requested them to return the following week. The patient was angry, responding that it was the GP's job to deal with whatever came, whenever it came. There was no human understanding of the doctor's situation.

Robin Downie has pointed out that such reflective work can help tune the physician's attention to nuances and hidden meanings in what patients say, as well as the ability to contextualise and connect – to carry over ideas and understandings from one situation to another.[28]

Clinical governance

As van Swanenberg and Harrison have pointed out, practitioners are coming increasingly under pressure to be accountable: 'clinicians [can] no longer live in isolation from themselves, their colleagues, or their patients. The arrival of clinical governance is a public recognition of that fact.'[29] A Royal College of Nursing report on clinical governance argues that it is 'fundamentally about developing an open learning culture that shares information, based on effective multi-professional team working.'[30] I would insert five more factors which, as well as information, should be shared: experience, knowledge, skills, feelings and ideas.

Bringing clinical issues, relationships and encounters into the open, and sharing them in the way outlined in this chapter, increases accountability; an open and honest examination or discussion of these elements can moreover greatly improve clinical quality, and enable continuous improvement.

A final story about misunderstanding from the same group:

Moira's story

Last time as I was printing out Jim's prescription, he interrupted my thoughts with a tentative 'I don't suppose you've any of those blue tablets, have you doctor?' 'Blue tablets' I mused looking at his notes 'blue tablets ... what's blue and in tablet form? Digoxin?', I queried. 'You're not on digoxin. Which blue tablets Jim?'

'You know, doctor,' he said meaningfully, 'you know those ones that everyone's talking about.' He shuffled in his seat in embarrassment.

'Oh,' I said as the penny dropped, 'Viagra ... oh, I'm sorry I didn't realise what you meant.'

The tentativeness was understandable, but the idea that I might be in possession of some nevertheless amused me. I imagined keeping a drawful of Viagra to give to my favoured male patients, or to give out like the stickers we give to children – 'I've been good at the doctor's to-day' – or like Smarties after a painful injection or procedure.

'No, I haven't any on me to day, Jim, but we'll have to see if it is possible for you to get some help in that direction. The thing is we're not allowed to prescribe Viagra willie-nilly. Sorry, I'll rephrase that – we're not allowed to give Viagra out to every Tom, Dick and ... What I mean is, we have to examine you and do some blood tests to see if you fit certain criteria, laid down by the Government.'

'Och, never mind this time, doc. Shall we talk about it next time I come?' I wonder if there will be a next time.

MOIRA

This story enabled the group to discuss the way that issues which patients find embarrassing can prevent them from being open with the doctor, therefore causing inevitable misunderstanding. The physician's alertness to the kinds of areas which cause embarrassment can lessen the likelihood of misunderstanding. The group were able to discuss what these were in their experience, and how they handle them.

They also shared a view that Viagra has opened certain issues up: men feel a bit more confident to be open now that Viagra has made it a slightly more acceptable problem, and one which might be readily treatable. Moira had no idea this man had problems in this area, but now she will be on the lookout for him wanting to discuss them in further consultations.

Conclusions

Here is Jack Coulehan again:

To teach *emotional resilience* requires that we in medical education focus actively on the recognition and articulation of students' compassion and the subtle and complex language of the emotions ... Teaching methods grounded in the *narrative nature of medical knowledge, the use of stories to develop the moral imagination, and the use of creative writing to promote empathic understanding* all foster a commitment to tenderness and steadiness in medical learning... within a framework of emotional resilience, detachment must be viewed as a serious risk that leads to undesirable consequences in practising medicine, rather than as a goal of medical education [my italics].[31]

Reflective practice writing and group work does more than foster empathic relationships with patients and colleagues. It enables:

▶ a rich dissemination of expertise, knowledge and experience
▶ a critical evaluation of professional practice in a supportive peer forum; increased confidence in professional practice
▶ stress relief by examining troublesome areas of practice
▶ increased understanding of the pressures and needs of peers
▶ identification, examination and evaluation of learning needs
▶ an increase in self-confidence, self-respect as well as pleasure in the writing and sharing.

Back in my youth, I remember the pop group The Animals singing:

> *I'm just a soul whose intentions are good*
> *Oh lord, please don't let me be misunderstood.*

Good intentions and expert clinical knowledge are not sufficient in the practice of a good physician. Education, like that offered by reflective practice writing, especially when allied to carefully facilitated group work, harnesses and increases intentions, skills and understandings. Clinical effectiveness and patient satisfaction will be much increased, and costs reduced. Reflective practice writing offers an excellent opportunity to learn lessons from experience, and avoid failure.

Notes and references

1 Department of Health. *An organisation with a memory: report on an expert group on learning from adverse events in the NHS.* London: The Stationery Office, 2000.
2 Milne AA. *The world of Pooh.* London: Metheun, 1958.

3 Hippocrates (trans. Chadwick J, Mann WN). *Hippocratic writings*. Middlesex: Penguin, 1950.

4 Carson R. Teaching ethics in the context of the medical humanities. *Journal of Medical Ethics* 1994;**20(4)**:235–8.

5 Bolton G. *Reflective practice writing for professional development*. London: Sage, 2000.

6 Bolton G. Stories at work: reflective writing for practitioners. *Lancet* 1999;**354**: 243–5. See also reference five.

7 See reference 6.

8 Frost C, King N. *'Physician heal thyself': the emotional demands of general practice*. Proceedings of the British Psychological Society's Occupational Psychology Conference; 2000 Jan 5–7; Brighton.

9 See reference 5.

10 More ES. Empathy as an hermeneutic practice. *Theoretical Medicine* 1996;**17**:243–54.

11 Frank A. Narratives of illness and care: why now? Paper presented at 'Narrative Matters: Personal Essays and the Making of Health Policy' seminar; March 2000; Virginia.

12 Goleman D. *Emotional intelligence: why it can matter more than IQ*. London: Bloomsbury, 1995.

13 See reference 10.

14 Balint E, Norrell JS. *Six minutes for the patient: interactions in general practice consultation*. London: Tavistock, 1973.

15 See reference 10.

16 Rogers C, Frieberg HJ. *Freedom to learn*. New York: Maxwell, 1994.

17 See reference 10.

18 Berger J. *A fortunate man: the story of a country doctor*. Middlesex: Penguin, 1969.

19 Coulehan J. Empathy, passion and imagination: a medical triptych. *Journal of Medical Humanities* 1997;**18**:99–110.

20 Coulehan J. Tenderness and steadiness: emotions in medical practice. *Literature and Medicine* 1995;**14**:222–36.

21 See reference 8.

22 See reference 19.

23 Evison R. Helping individuals manage emotional responses. In: Payne RL, Cooper CL (eds). *Emotions at work: theory, research and applications in management*. London: Wiley and Sons (in press).

24 See reference 23.

25 Pennebaker JW, Kiecolt Glaser J, Glaser R. Disclosures of trauma and immune function: health implications for psychotherapy. *Journal of Consultative and Clinical Psychology* 1988;**56**:239–45.

26 Smyth JM, *et al.* Effects of writing about stressful experiences on symptom

reduction in patients with asthma or rheumatoid arthritis: a randomised trial. *Journal of the American Medical Association* 1999;**281**:1328–9.

27 Horder J. *I believe...* Proceedings of the Royal College of Physicians of Edinburgh; 1996;**26**:466–71.

28 Downie R. *Education.* Talk given to the Centre for Arts and Humanities in Health Care; June 2000; Durham.

29 van Swanenberg T, Harrison J. *Clinical governance in primary care.* London: Radcliffe Medical Press, 2000.

30 Royal College of Nursing. *Clinical governance: how can nurses get involved?* London: RCN, 2000.

31 See reference 20.

Acknowledgements

I would like to thank Debbie Kirklin for sending me off on this particularly enjoyable writing quest. I would like to thank all the practitioners with whom I have worked over the last fifteen years. In particular I thank Moira Brimacombe, Jo Cannon, Charles Heatley, Jane Searle, Caroline Walton, Rosie Welch, Shirley Brierley, Clare Connolly, Maggie Eisner, Seth Jenkinson, Sheena McCain, Mark Purvis, Becky Ship and Mike Leuty (and Mike for pointing out the Pooh quote to me). It has been a constant adventure of discovery for me, alongside these inquisitive, adventurous and generous clinicians.

CHAPTER NINE

A 'necessary Inhumanity'?
The role of detachment in medical practice

Ruth Richardson

The eighteenth century surgeon-anatomist William Hunter urged his students to gain '*A necessary Inhumanity*' by dissecting the dead.[1] Hunter knew that trainee doctors could not be too tender, and that this inhumanity would stand his students in good stead in dealing with the surgery of the day, which – before anaesthesia, antisepsis and blood transfusion – needed to be not only accurate but fast if it was to be successful.

Nowadays, we call this necessary inhumanity 'clinical detachment' or something similar which sounds less emotive, more scientific. But in a sense Hunter's words are more honest. They help clarify what he was actually urging – inhumanity – but only to a necessary degree. The phrase has more precision, a suggestion of calibration, even a hint of warning, which 'clinical detachment' or 'clinical objectivity' lack.

Whatever we call it, it clearly has value even today: it can protect both patient and doctor, allowing each generation to learn how to examine, to diagnose, to treat, to operate, and to verify diagnoses after death. It's key, then. But there are also dangers.

A doctor currently practising in the UK recalls:

I'm [glad] to recall my memories of the dissection room ... to lay a few old ghosts. Dissecting earthworms in biology was no preparation .... To avoid disgracing myself on the first day (I was rather a sensitive soul, and if someone pricked their finger I was the one who needed the brandy) my friend and I stole up to the dissection room during the summer holidays, where there were perhaps twenty tables with corpses on, covered by greasy canvas sheets. We gingerly lifted up the corner of one these sheets to see what was underneath ... [The advance visit] meant that we could walk into the dissection room on the first day of term with our heads held high, and a great air of bravado, having steeled ourselves. One of the students was unable to sit through the introductory lecture, which was about scalpels and forceps, and fat and fascia, because of the thought of dissecting. And the first week that we were in the dissecting room, he spent throwing up in the loo. At the end of the first week he blew his brains out with a shotgun.

The experience of dissecting was a strange way to be introduced to patients. In Jewish medical schools, for example, they start by going out to look at the medical system on a kibbutz, whereas ... we start with a pickled patient. And this curious introduction resulted in such misbehaviour as games of cricket played with human arms and large blood-clots. Even shy and gentle me looked down one day to see that I was swinging a human head nonchalantly by its windpipe.[2]

This passage conveys an understanding – a rather painful one – of the impact of a conventional medical training. This doctor is still haunted by it. He describes his younger self as fearful of exposing his own sensitivity, and remembers the calamitous effect on a contemporary who could not endure the experience. This doctor reveals the astonishment he felt when he realised that against all the odds, he had somehow acquired a detachment which apparently extended to his own arm: '*Even shy and gentle me looked down one day to see ....*'

This young man acquired an altered sense-perception of his own actions, and began to treat the dead with indifference (not to say animosity) with remarkable rapidity. This was his first step on the lowest rung of the professional ladder, his first lesson at medical school. He himself has likened the experience to battle exposure. Both the dead and the living were its victims.

Of course, dissection is not the only brutalising part in the process of becoming a doctor. Attending postmortems (especially on patients one has known in life) and the punishing period of sleep deprivation caused by excessive hours laden with the stress of heavy responsibility (the common experience of house jobs) often equals or exceeds it in doctors' estimation. But until recently dissection was always the first to which young people were exposed, and for centuries the dissection room has been used as a threshold or liminal space, its activity as a kind of rite of passage, through which ordinary young people are transformed into initiates of the mysteries of the medical life.

History offers a long term context for individual experiences of medical training. An awareness of the history of health care in the context of our society might assist self-reflection – might help keep initiates in touch with the wider culture they have been induced to leave, might help them remain humane despite the bruising process of training. Of course many doctors manage this without assistance, retaining something of their pre-medical values. The doctor I've quoted suffered a sort of existential unease at what he'd been forced to undergo, and took a conscious decision to deal with it at an early stage:

> I found myself looking at the body as a wonderful machine, but not as a creature with a soul – that worried me a bit. What in fact I had to do was consciously unlearn that sort of thing, and start to look at human beings as human beings.

This doctor speaks very simply, and I think rather downplays the importance of what he's saying, but what he's describing is fundamental to humane medicine.

I once attended a weekend course given by a Hollywood screenwriter, who shared with the class all his tips for structuring and developing a film-script. I was fascinated to find films dissected, specimen sequences extracted for exhibition, even cloned for study. One of the key messages was the importance of the 'backstory': the tale from the past which invariably emerges somewhere near the beginning of every film, providing the key to the motivation of the main protagonist, and sometimes, the key to the resolution of the entire film.

The acquisition of clinical detachment is a backstory in every doctor's biography, and in every clinical encounter. Every doctor has a backstory, and so does every patient. So too does every medical discipline. I suspect that much of this goes unacknowledged, and that 'clinical detachment' often works as a barrier between doctors and patients, to the detriment of all.

Three episodes from the past illustrate the potential for inhumanity in clinical detachment. Each has implications for the present moment in the history of health care.

Drug budgets

In the midsummer of 1872 a London doctor was appointed Medical Officer at the Westminster Workhouse. He was conducted around the building by the man who had held the post for the previous forty years, Mr French.

Poor Law contracts of employment ruled that all medicines dispensed to workhouse patients were to be paid for out of the doctor's salary. The contract was designed to control the national drugs budget. In the course of this tour Mr French laughingly confided his trade secret, that he pocketed all his salary by means of the simple expedient of giving no physic. All patients – whatever their condition, or suffering, and whether in mild, severe or even mortal pain – were treated with coloured peppermint-water.

Since his nurse never had any medicine to give, she frankly admitted that she'd not troubled herself about the patients, such was the influence of the doctor in this institution. She was about to learn her duties.

French does not seem to have grasped the character of his successor, or he might have kept his own counsel. The new man was Dr Joseph Rogers, a doctor with extensive workhouse experience, who was later to describe the encounter – and name French – in his *Reminiscences*.[3]

Originally from a Hampshire medical family, Rogers was a qualified apothecary and surgeon, who had set up in general practice in Dean Street, Soho, in 1844.[4] The district was badly affected by the cholera epidemic of 1854–5 – the famously contaminated Broad Street pump was just up the road. Most of Rogers' paying patients either died or moved away, and he found his living gone, in a district with an unhealthy reputation. So he competed for and obtained the only salaried work available: medical officer at the local workhouse, a few blocks further north in Cleveland Street. The building still exists, and is now the outpatients' department of the Middlesex Hospital.

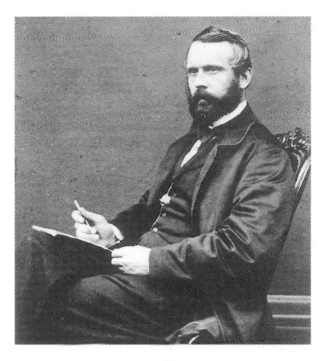

Dr Joseph Rogers

The Strand Union Workhouse was worse than anything described by Dickens. Illness, insanity and old age were then the primary causes of poverty, and Rogers found himself responsible for nearly five hundred sick and dying patients throughout the building. Only eight per cent of the inmates were judged to be medically well. Rogers had to work in grossly insanitary conditions, and in such overcrowding that patients could only get out at the ends of their beds. Epidemics of measles and fevers resulted in more deaths than recoveries.

Rogers was expected to treat all the sick under his care in this huge hell-hole of an old hospital, out of his wages of £50 a year. He later observed that 'the provision of ... medicines [to the sick people in the workhouse] was to me in every sense a pecuniary loss'. The method of remuneration appealed to and benefited the worst motives of unscrupulous doctors – while penalising well-motivated and benevolent ones. Rogers saw it as doubly pernicious: corrupting and brutalizing doctors while exacerbating the suffering of the sick and dying.

So what do Mr French and Dr Rogers have to do with us, today? With the help of the *Lancet*, Rogers campaigned against the 'gross abuse' of

113

penalising workhouse doctors for prescribing proper treatments.[5]
The Poor Law administration was eventually shamed into establishing
a system of capitation payment for salary, with a separate dedicated
drugs budget – which remains the basis of remuneration for general
practitioners in the National Health Service.

Rogers was later sacked from the Strand Union Workhouse for
defending standards of patient care, and used his freedom to campaign
for better conditions for the sick poor and their medical attendants by
founding the Association for the Improvement of London Workhouse
Infirmaries, and the Poor Law Medical Officers' Association. These
campaigning bodies were so successful that by the 1890s twenty new
hospitals (10,000 new beds) had been opened for London's sick poor.
Many of these hospital buildings are still in use: millions of Londoners
(like me) have been born or treated in them.

Imagine the sense of déja vu, when I recently found a report in a copy
of the medical newspaper *Pulse* concerning current debate about ageism
in the NHS, access to expensive medicines, and balancing practice
remuneration against the costs of prescribing. The report quoted
Dr Anne Dyson, a Chelmsford GP, as saying:

> We have made as many savings as we can without cutting into patient care.
> The flesh was cut right back to the bone a long time ago. How can we be
> unbiased in prescribing when you know it might come out of your pocket?[6]

Presuming upon consent

Transplantation is often presented as a phenomenon of the twentieth
century. In fact it's a development in the much longer history of
surgery, which is itself rooted in anatomical exploration. Looking back
at that history, with an awareness of the current shortage of organs for
transplant, one cannot help but perceive that the problems of the past
are being played out afresh in our own time.

This eighteenth century cartoon[7] shows a surgeon dentist and his
assistant, transplanting teeth for wealthy elderly clients. A notice
announces 'Most Money Given for Live Teeth': the usual supply was
obtained by graverobbers from the mouths of the dead.[8]

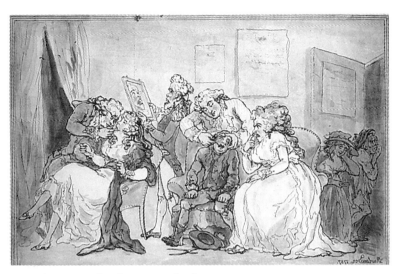

Transplanting teeth (Thomas Rowlandson).

As the cartoon shows, transplantation has strong antecedents in the eighteenth century, traceable to the surgeon-anatomist John Hunter (brother of William, he of the 'necessary Inhumanity'). John trained under William, and both ran anatomy schools in central London, with dissecting tables supplied by body snatchers. Both were avid specimen collectors for their own museums. William specialised in what we now call obstetrics, John in general and experimental surgery.

John Hunter performed successful auto-transplants on cockerels, moving the spur from a bird's heel to its own head, where it proliferated. It was only a short step to the practical application of such ideas on human subjects. In the 1770s, he recommended the transplantation of teeth, and it was rapidly adopted by high-class dentists.

Among the first to expose the exploitative nature of these operations was Helenus Scott, whose novel *Adventures of a rupee* appeared anonymously in 1782. It revealed the catastrophic long-term effects on children already poor, of the removal of healthy second teeth: the dietary impact of being unable to masticate, and the permanent damage to facial appearance, resulting in the likely loss of a normal married or working life.[9]

The cartoon, by Thomas Rowlandson, was first published in 1790 – in the immediate aftermath of the French Revolution. Its fierce censure was directed at both the wealthy beneficiaries of the operation and their assiduous agents, the surgeons. Both are shown as vain and contemptible exploiters of poverty. Rowlandson's dental surgeon advertises his social pretensions with a warrant: 'Dentist to her High Mightyness the Empress of Russia'. The 'donors', if you can call them that, are very poor children: the lad whose teeth are being extracted in the centre is a chimney sweep's climbing boy, the others are in rags. The girl holding her jaw gazes at the small coin she's been paid for her newly erupted second set.

The demise of the practice can be traced not to ethical questionability, but to clinical failure – it was rarely a long term success and decomposition of the tooth invariably followed after a time. Worse still, the physician Sir William Watson, Vice President of the Royal Society, went public in 1785 in the *Medical Transactions* of the Royal College of Physicians, describing a case in which syphilis was transmitted to a recipient with an infected tooth, leading to a horrible death.[10]

How any doctor could have failed to recognise the long-term damage to a child I fail to see, especially Hunter, who wrote a book on the natural history of human teeth[11] and who executed exquisite work on the anatomy of childhood dentition for his museum. Yet Hunter was apparently impervious to lay ethical criticism. Despite mounting evidence, he continued to deny clinical failure, and to cast doubt on stories of disease spread. I've occasionally seen the cockerel mentioned as a progenitor of modern transplantation, and Hunter is often referred to as the 'father of modern surgery', but the story of the teeth seems often to have been unaccountably overlooked.[12]

The inhumanity in this story speaks for itself, and its implications for today both worry and reassure. Let me explain: in 1999 the British Medical Association voted to recommend to government a policy of 'presumed consent' in organ procurement. Fortunately – and it was this I found reassuring – the Department of Health responded swiftly to the BMA's deeply retrogressive recommendation, publishing the results of a recent survey showing little public support for the idea, and stating firmly that it does not intend to change the present system of freely consented donation.

Dissection and transplantation have deep roots in similar soil: the history of one illuminates the other. Doctors have always found legal limits on access to the dead inadequate and restrictive, and they repeatedly found alternative, illegal sources. Until 1832 the only legal source of corpses for dissection was the gallows – not enough bodies were available, which is why for centuries we had bodysnatching, and eventually murder, for anatomy.[13] The Anatomy Act of 1832 requisitioned instead the bodies of people too poor to pay for their own burial: paupers dying in hospitals and workhouses – the very folk whom Mr French denied physic. The Anatomy Act is still in force, but is pretty much a dead letter, because it in turn provoked such bitter opposition and non-compliance as to cause ongoing chronic shortage.

The problem of shortage existed – apparently dogged by the irresolvable obstacle of public hostility – from the mediaeval era to the mid twentieth century. Public antipathy to dissection has since subsided sufficiently to provide adequate supplies. Only since the era of the National Health Service have there been sufficient bodies available, without public opposition or controversy, given freely by publicly spirited citizens.[14]

As well as whole body donors, and blood donors, over eight million British citizens have currently registered themselves on the UK organ donor register, established less than a decade ago. These phenomena suggest that there exists among the British public a significant fund of goodwill towards medical endeavour, which it would be deeply foolish to squander.

Recent events have revealed, however, a profound asymmetry in UK health care. The NHS is paid for by the public. Generous donations are made by members of the public to help train new doctors, and to help other patients in the system – whole bodies, organs, blood. We have trusted our doctors – we have had faith – but recent revelations concerning the secret removal of organs and tissues from children ('presumed consent' in earnest, indeed), and their secret disposal as 'clinical waste', proclaims that the public's good faith has been met with bad.[15]

The BMA might have achieved more and acted in better faith towards the public, had its meeting voted for a mass signing of organ donor cards before television cameras. After all, what is more honest, to offer oneself as a donor, or to presume, or force, someone else to perform that duty?

Specimen taking

My last example concerns specimen taking directly, both for museums and for research. Like other medical museums with historic origins, the Hunterian Museum, at the Royal College of Surgeons in London, provides a fossil record of the procurement policies of past specimen collectors. Named after its founder, John Hunter, by far the great majority of the human specimens on display there were taken without consent, from gallows, graves, or during surgical operations or postmortems.

Presuming upon the consent of the public – or assuming it to be altogether unnecessary – has been almost an orthodoxy in the disciplines of anatomy and pathology since their inception. These unconsented exhibits are epitomised by the great skeleton of the 'Irish Giant', Charles O'Brien, who was almost eight feet tall. In the 1780s he was a human exhibit – rather like the Elephant Man. He caused a sensation wherever he displayed himself, and was able to earn good

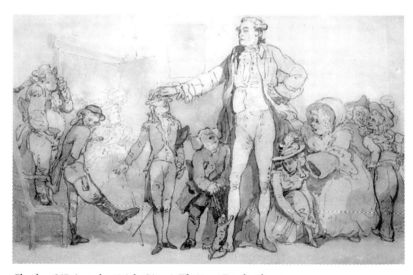

Charles O'Brien, the 'Irish Giant' (Thomas Rowlandson).

amounts of money. He knew the doctors would want his skeleton for their museums, but wished so fiercely to protect himself from dissection that shortly before he died in 1783 O'Brien left a large sum of money (said to be £500) to ensure that his body be buried at sea in a lead coffin. His undertaker, however, was heavily bribed (apparently to the same amount) to deliver the corpse instead to John Hunter's dissection rooms.[16] The victim of this spectacular theft still stands to this day in a great glass case at the heart of the Royal College of Surgeons' Museum. O'Brien's skeleton serves as a monument to the morality of the medical museum, a monument to theft, to medical acquisitiveness, to an historic injustice. It was from the deep basement of this institution that the artist Anthony Noël Kelly took the body parts which recently landed him in gaol for theft.[17] The irony of his prosecution cannot be lost on anyone who contemplates the sources of the College's specimen collection.

The originally conjoined disciplines of anatomy and pathology have diverged since Hunter's day. Yet pathology as a discipline – and its customary manner of specimen taking, too – has preserved many of the attitudes of its forbears, as well as those who served under the ethos of the Anatomy Act.

Many hundreds, possibly thousands of parents in Bristol, Liverpool, Southampton, Leeds, London and elsewhere have suffered profound distress because their children's organs have been 'retained' without consent after postmortem/autopsy. It is only a matter of time before the general public becomes aware that the practice has never been confined to infants.

I have interviewed some of the parents caught up in this tragedy, and have found that roughly half of them would have been willing to donate their child's heart if it might have saved other parents' grief ... but they were not asked. Had the doctors respected these dead children and their bereft parents enough to ask permission before ransacking their little bodies, there might have been half the number available, and moreover neither scandal, nor hurt. Of course, this is only a rough and ready computation, based on an opportunistic series of interviews with a small sample of parents. Nevertheless, it's clear that the attempt to maximise yield by deception has caused terrible anguish and damage to bereaved relatives and has brought the entire medical profession into disrepute.

I'm a rationalist. I have no difficulty with the idea that medical science needs body parts, that bodies need to be dissected, that students need to train, that surgeons need to understand foetal and other abnormalities, that postmortem findings are important. But I also believe that human beings have feelings, and it is the job of a caring profession to care for feelings. We all have rights, and one of the most fundamental of human rights is the right of self-determination.

This scandal reveals an inhumane attitude of mind which has pervaded medical dealings with the public. Because we have feelings, because we experience sorrow, and because some of us don't relish the process of allowing unfamiliar people to interfere, much less quarry, the bodies of our relatives, the medical profession seems to regard us as 'other' – emotional, stupid, ignorant, unscientific *and* easily duped. Medical professionals cannot pretend that only pathologists are responsible: surgeons, nurses, hospital and mortuary staff, coroners, even some general practitioners, have known about it for years. The attitude is inhumane because it denies our common humanity, and I suspect may derive from the fact that many doctors learn in the process of becoming doctors, to deny their own.

As we've seen, it's quite possible for doctors to behave inhumanely – Mr French laughed as he described the coloured water he'd meted out to the dying for forty years; John Hunter extracted healthy teeth from the mouths of poor children, and paid the undertaker to deny the Irish Giant his rightful burial. These doctors were without pity, able to ignore, deny, overlook or even despise their patients' humanity. Their motives were fundamentally acquisitive. Their activities thrived in closed institutions – the workhouse, the dental surgery, the anatomy school. In all these stories, too, local and national government had a hand – failing to protect children, administering a heartless Poor Law, choosing neither to oversee nor adequately to regulate the conduct of the anatomy school, the dentist's surgery, the workhouse, the modern hospital and its pathology lab, or the coroner's mortuary.

Each of these stories also has its humane medical professional, who nudged matters towards change – Dr Rogers, serving his workhouse patients even to the extent of losing his job; Sir William Watson, lifting the lid on a corrupt and highly lucrative surgical intervention by revealing its clinical consequences; and Dr Stephen Bolsin, who blew the whistle at Bristol.

In each case, the humane doctor's moral intelligence has been more in touch with public opinion than has the inhumane, which I think tells us something also about the essential decency of the ordinary people of this country. And in each case, public opinion, and members of the lay public, have been vital in promoting reform. Rogers received the active support of Charles Dickens, Florence Nightingale, and hundreds of others who were less well-known; Watson's criticisms were subsequent to those of Helenus Scott and Thomas Rowlandson; the Bristol parents and the national press have been at the heart of the movement to bring about the long-delayed reform of pathology.

I've argued that the term 'necessary Inhumanity' more accurately describes the alienation required of doctors in some circumstances, than do modern, sanitized coinages such as 'clinical detachment'. 'Detachment' and 'objectivity' imply separation, not engagement: creating distance not only from patients, but from the self. The process may well be required, but where it becomes too extreme or prolonged, it can damage everybody, including donors, family members, doctors themselves, and the wider society. Somehow, the good doctor manages to hold on to, or consciously acquire, a necessary *humanity*.[18]

A 'necessary Inhumanity' is in my view a greatly preferable term for the process of learning the necessary distance the trainee doctor must develop to become a good clinician. It is preferable because it more honestly and precisely describes an aspect of the doctor–patient relationship.

Were we to resurrect the term, to consciously return to using it, knowing what we know, and with the science we now have, it might become evident that clinical detachment is not a simple acquisition, but a spectrum of sensibility which can range from extreme cruelty to conscious empathy. Most of us are able to discern that Nazi doctors were off one end of the scale, but it is also important to be aware that so too is some of the behaviour in our own country, institutionalised in our own health service, even in our own time.

The notion of a necessary inhumanity could be valuable because the questions it prompts might serve as an effective calibrator: How 'necessary' in these circumstances? For how long? And with *what effect*? Resurrecting and knowingly re-embracing the term 'inhumanity' *now* might mean an awareness of its dangerous potential, which in turn might mean there'd be less *of* it about.

Acknowledgements

This is an edited version of a talk given at the conference *The Healing Arts: the role of the humanities in medical education*, at the Royal Society of Arts, London 30th March 2000. An abbreviated version was subsequently published in *Medical Humanities* December 2000.[19] I thank Brian Hurwitz and Deborah Kirklin for their helpful observations on this piece.

The photograph of Dr Joseph Rogers in this chapter is reproduced by kind permission of the Bodleian Library, University of Oxford (Thorold Rogers Box 8). The two illustrations by Thomas Rowlandson are reproduced by kind permission of the President and Council of the Royal College of Surgeons of England.

A Victorian student contemplates humanity

Ruth Richardson and Brian Hurwitz

This is a fine piece of creative writing by a Victorian medical student, which appeared anonymously in 1893 as a small shilling pamphlet, printed by Adlard and Son of Bartholomew Close. It tells a remarkable story, illuminating in a unique way a dissecting room and its inhabitants at the turn of the nineteenth century. A desultory student who has treated the dead body on which he has been working with some carelessness, if not with disrespect, has a remarkable experience which causes him to resolve to behave differently henceforth. The story suggests that early stages of medical training can play powerfully on an initiate's subconsciousness.

This version[20] is a distillation of the original text, given where possible in the author's own words. Summary passages in square brackets are ours. Elisions have not been individually noted. The piece is followed by a brief discussion; superscript letters indicate commentary notes (p131).

It was a raw frosty evening of the 31st December 18–. Before the fire in a small, dingy sitting-room, of a typical lodging house in Middleton Square, sat a young medical student.[A] He was tall, and of prepossessing appearance; twenty-four years of age, and was pursuing his studies – but had not got very close to them – at St Bartholomew's Hospital. His name as it usually figured in the charge sheet was Henry Trottingham Carlton, but he was known to his intimates as 'Tubby'.

Tubby was lying before the fire of his unpretentious sitting-room that evening, meditating upon things in general and upon the likelihood of his being ploughed for his 'second college' in January.[B] Tubby had not been home for Christmas. He had written to his parents, and informed them that he could not possibly spare the time, as the examination was so close at hand. His father, by way of consolation, had sent him a five-pound note, which the directors of the Alhambra had undertaken to look after for him.[C] So on this particular evening Tubby felt disconsolate, and wished that some good fairy would drop in and present him with sufficient money wherewith to see the old year out in a manner befitting a medical student.

Being thoroughly weary of his new game – which consisted in shutting his eyes, while he removed the carpal bones one by one from his right trowser pocket and placed them in his left, endeavouring to 'spot' them in transit[D] – he decided that he would go down to the Hospital to see if he could find anybody about who would cheer him up a bit and, perhaps, he thought, be induced to lend him a trifle.

[He enters the precinct whistling the music hall song 'The Man Who Broke the Bank at Monte Carlo'. The place is deserted. Seeking in vain for anyone to ask for a loan, he hears voices across the square towards the medical college. He goes over in search of a pal.]

A curious ray of light [proceeded] *from what he knew to be a trap-door,*[E] *through which material destined for the future advancement of science was carried, previous to being titivated up, in order to present as respectable an appearance as was consistent with the probability of making their first appearance in public in the 'lithotomy' position.*[F]

[Tubby knows that the dissecting room attendant is away until the New Year, so not without some trepidation, he goes down to investigate. He is astonished to find that he is one of a company.]

Tubby recognised them at once by their copper-coloured skins and their shaven heads. They were all of the male sex and apparently advanced in years as well as in odour, and were all in a state of nudity bordering upon the indecent.[G] *They seemed somewhat surprised to see Tubby there, but beyond staring at him in a rather rude way, they did not molest him.*

They all made for the dissecting-room door as if moved by a common impulse, while Tubby followed, wondering, in their rear. Tubby was instantly stopped by a portly individual who demanded his ticket.

[There is an altercation, in which the student has to admit he has no ticket, and the door-keeper endeavours to keep him out.]

A fat dilapidated man who had been attracted by the noise came over to the door in order to see what was the matter.

You can imagine Tubby's astonishment when he recognised this man as the very fat individual upon whose leg he had been experimenting for the last three weeks. We say 'experimenting' because all Tubby's work in the rooms partook rather of the nature of experiments, inasmuch as he worked upon no recognised methods. The orthodox manner is to begin with Scarpa's triangle, and so on, working gradually and methodically down the leg.[H] *But Tubby did differently. When he felt any curiosity with regard to the whereabouts of any particular nerve or artery, he would select the spot under which he supposed the object of his research to lie, and would dig a hole there and commence to hunt. If he found the nerve or artery in question, which he never did by any chance if it happened to be smaller in diameter than his little finger, he became uproariously happy. If, on the other hand, he was baffled – which he frequently was – he concluded that the man had not got the article, and was perfectly contented.*

Well, Tubby not only recognised this man, but the man instantly knew Tubby, and what was more, appeared to be extremely pleased to see him. He shook Tubby heartily by the hand.

'It's all right, doorkeeper,' said he, 'this gentleman is a friend of mine.'

'Come along, Mr Carlton,' said the fat man as he seized Tubby by the arm, 'permit me to constitute your host for this evening.'

'You are very good,' murmured Tubby, somewhat bewildered. 'Well I am blowed!'

This remark escaped Tubby quite unconsciously, and was called forth by the extraordinary spectacle that met his gaze when entering the room. It was brilliantly lighted. In each fireplace roared a seductive-looking fire.[I] Seated around the well-known tables, which were loaded with beverages of every description, were some two or three hundred people. They were quite naked; indeed, some had gone one better than this and had parted with some of their skin and superficial fascia. It was certainly a most astounding spectacle.

When Tubby had recovered from his first shock of surprise, he began to feel rather uncomfortable – this time not from fear, but rather from a feeling of annoyance. If there was one thing in the world that Tubby disliked more than another it was eccentricity. Now, knowing this about Tubby, you can readily imagine how extremely upset he was, as he perceived at once that an individual in a lounge suit was singularly out of place among this assembly.

He felt this so keenly, and showed his annoyance so unmistakably in his countenance that his elderly friend divining the cause, suggested that he should step into the prosector's room and remove his clothing.[J] Tubby brightened up at this idea, observing at once a ready solution of the difficulty. He took his protector's advice, and emerged thence shortly afterwards, resplendent in nature's uniform: somewhat embarrassed perhaps at first, but still, on the whole, much preferring it to his former costume.

'Come along, Sir,' said his fat friend, 'let us get a seat at the Chairman's table.'[K]

'Right you are,' said Tubby, 'but I wish that you would tell me what it's all about. What is the meaning of this gathering?'

'Well', replied the fat man, 'for the last ten years we have held a social gathering here on 31st December, to celebrate the entry of the New Year, and to have a little social intercourse generally. You see it is only once a year that we meet our old friends. These gatherings were inaugurated in order to promote good fellowship. We used to meet in the post-mortem room, but soon after we had started, and the chaps got to know of it, the function became so popular that we were obliged to seek a larger apartment.'[L]

'But surely,' said Tubby, 'all these people are not from this Hospital?'

'Oh! dear no!' replied his friend. 'We welcome anybody. Most of us have friends at other hospitals, and they generally come over to see us on the day.'

'Who is the gentleman in the chair?' inquired Tubby, 'I seem to recognise him.'

'Most certainly you do, Mr Carlton', said the fat man. 'The gentleman in the chair is our worthy President. I have no doubt but that during ordinary days you have observed him suspended from an elevated position, over by that pillar yonder.'

'Why, he is the painted skeleton!' exclaimed Tubby.

[Tubby discovers that he has missed the evening's discussion, on cremation and its probable consequences upon the welfare of the community represented by the gathering.^M The Chairman rises to address the company]:

'Gentlemen,' said he, 'we are gathered together once more under this hospitable roof, in order to hold our annual soirée, which, for the benefit of those of you who have not received a French education, I would mention means "evening" from a social point of view (hear, hear).^N I see many old and esteemed faces around me this evening, and also some new ones' (Cheers).

[The Chairman welcomes newcomers, and accepts apologies for absence from an individual unavoidably detained awaiting a post-mortem, who is anxious to assist in the discovery of the cause of his own death by not adding any confounding signs as a result of social indulgence. The Chairman observes to cheers that such a conscientious personage will be a credit to their community.^O He calls upon Mr Pneumonia Tertius for a song. Tubby asks his friend about the singer's name.]

'When we join this community we drop our former names, and receive the name of the disease from which we are supposed to have died. The gentleman died of pneumonia, but as there were already two of the same name senior to him, we call him 'Tertius'.^P

'How do you manage,' inquired Tubby, 'when the cause of death has not been ascertained?'

'We call them "Neurotic",' said his friend. 'We have lots of them here. Occasionally we get most complicated people. Take myself, for instance. I was sent in as "Typhoid", treated for "Meningitis", and died from the bursting of an "Aneurysm of the Abdominal Aorta".'

No further conversation was possible owing to the thunderous applause which greeted Pneumonia Tertius upon his rising to sing.

[His song is a parody of the Policeman's Song from the *Pirates of Penzance*]:

Pneumonia Tertius's song

When a human dies, folk usually consider
                                  'Ly consider.
That he's better off when planted in a hole;
                                  In a hole.
The contract goes out to the lowest bidder,
                                  Lowest bidder.
They never trouble much about his soul,
                                  'Bout his soul.
Everybody thinks they've done their duty,
                                  Done their duty.
When a stone's inscribed in laudatory terms;
                                  'Datory terms.
Then they leave him to develop symptoms fruity,
                                  Symptoms fruity.
In the questionable company of worms,
                                  Of worms.
Taking one consideration with another,
                                  With another.
A planted corpse is not a happy one.
                                  Happy one.
How different is the case with us, my brothers
                                  Oh, my brothers.
We become, when dead, most valuable stock;
                                  'Able stock.
We make a fresh appearance 'long with others,
                                  'Long with others.
In a dignified position on a block.
                                  On a block.
We're cut up in a systematic manner,
                                  'Matic manner.
And not devoid of scientific skill;
                                  'Tific skill.
Our limbs are wrapped in towels that cost a tanner,
                                  Cost a tanner.
The 'rooms' are warmed to guard us from a chill.
                                  From a chill.

Taking one consideration with another,

With another.

We've got the 'pull' on any planted corpse.

Planted corpse.[Q]

The song was greeted with loud and continued applause.

[The Chairman then calls for another song, but unfortunately the next singer],

Mr Carcinoma was not capable of very distinct articulation, somebody having clipped one of his superior maxillary bones into two or three pieces.

[Only the chorus was audible]:

Carcinoma's chorus

As I strut about the rooms so fine
With my independent air,
And my head devoid of hair,
Oh, I look so debonair.
The ladies say I am so sly,
And the fellows look with a jealous eye
On the man who died of rectal carcinoma.[R]

[Afterwards, Tubby's friend rises to say a few words].

He only wished to remark that in his opinion the company ought to feel very honoured by the presence of the distinguished guest on his right (loud cheers). He begged to propose Mr Carlton's health (loud and prolonged cheers).

[In turn, Tubby rises to answer]:

'Gentlemen,' said he, 'No words of mine can convey to you the feeling of pleasure that is within me at being allowed to take part tonight in your annual festival (cheers). I assure you, gentlemen, that had I known of your gathering in previous years I should not only have attended myself, but I should have brought a few friends with me. I feel deeply that we students have a great deal to learn from you in the way of organising social evenings (loud cheers). Our smoking concert club is the only affair that we possess that appeals to everybody and offers a welcome to all (cheers). Of course we are scorned by the aristocrats of the senior musical clubs, but we do not mind this. We know that it is against all precedent to cater for the insignificant student, the pitiful first and second year's man.[S] *I can assure you, gentlemen, that the smoking concert club will be delighted to see any of you who care to come to it' (cheers).*[T]

'Before I sit down, gentlemen, I should like to again thank you for your most excellent entertainment, and to wish you every success in the New Year (cheers). I also wish to propose a toast, and that is to the Chairman (loud cheers). I was presented to him some years ago by Mr J— (cheers), and have renewed the acquaintance upon several occasions.[U] But I must candidly confess that from the cursory inspection that I made of him, as he dangled from his iron bracket, I did not dream for a moment that he was such a worthy gentleman. I give you the health of the Chairman' (loud and prolonged cheers, the whole audience rising).

When the excitement had subsided, the Chairman rose to reply.

[He thanks the company for the toast, and invites Tubby to return the following year].

'While hanging from my bracket, gentlemen, I see many things, which naturally you, who are as a rule in the horizontal position, are unable to observe. And from the great length of time that I have been in these rooms, and the number of students who annually pass through them, you will readily believe that I have been the silent witness of many a curious scene.

'Mr Carlton, I am glad to inform you, is most assiduous in his attendance here (cheers). Times out of number I have known him to spend nearly twenty minutes of his valuable time in our company during the day (cheers). His favourite position is before the fire (laughter). Nay, this is no laughing matter, gentlemen, when you consider what this means: the sacrifice to clothing and health that a warm at the dissecting-room fire entails. Mr Carlton, I have no doubt, will bear me out when I say, that a quarter of an hour in front of our remarkable fire means a new pair of trowsers and an acute attack of tonsillitis (loud laughter). Of course you are done with trowsers and tonsillitis, gentlemen (hear, hear).

'As you see by the clock that it only wants five minutes to twelve, it is absolutely imperative that I should stop. My best wishes to you, gentlemen, for the New Year, and may we celebrate this day for many years to come (loud and prolonged cheers). Just at this moment the clock struck twelve,[V] and as the first strokes of the gong echoed through the rooms, the company mounted the different tables, and crossing their arms, they grasped the hands of their neighbours on either side. Thus they waited until the clock had finished striking. Then, at a signal from the Chairman they emitted a mighty and glass shattering cheer, and then broke off into the following version of Auld Lang Syne:

And now my lads, before we part,
With friendship in our hearts,
We'll give our Chairman three times three,

And one for good old Bart's.
And yet another for our club,
We're men of many parts,
We still can stand upright awhile,
For the sake of good old Bart's.[W]

When they had finished, they cheered again and again, and having wished each other all the compliments of the season, they began to depart in as orderly a manner as could be expected. About seventy of them insisted upon going in the lift at the same time, others wanted to burn the tables, another detachment wanted to go round the wards and frighten the patients.[X] But on the whole they were quite representative of the ordinary crowd of humans when departing from a function. Tubby and his host took affectionate leave of each other – Tubby promising to treat that gentleman's leg in future in a more respectful manner.'[Y]

[Tubby finds to his horror that the prosector's room is locked, and is ejected from the building by the officious doorkeeper. Profoundly embarrassed by his own nakedness, he races away out of the Hospital precinct and across Smithfield, and in his anxious flight, trips and falls. He finds himself being awoken from his sleep on the floor beside the fire by his landlady, who has ventured into his room to wish him a Happy New Year. They part, having exchanged kind wishes for the year to come].

Discussion

First reactions to the dissecting room and to dissection may include faintness, physical symptoms of unease, even flight. Anxiety may be expressed as embarrassment, levity, or bravado. Coping mechanisms include the bestowal by students of fictitious names, speculative personalities or life stories upon bodies on the slab. A curious sort of bond can develop between the student and the 'person' of the dead body. The emotional experience contrasts with and supplements students' efforts to internalize anatomical knowledge. There may evolve a sense of familiarity, contact, intimacy, of transgression, invasion, perhaps guilt, and obligation.[21,22,23,24]

In this dream-tale is embedded the author's own wishful thinking: the dead not only have names, but personalities, and even active and interesting private lives of their own. They are not passive victims of student ineptitude and maltreatment. Rather than annoyance or anger, they exhibit friendship, forgiveness and humour towards the student.

In its own way, this tale implies that beyond the student's first rite of passage, lies another: a more internalized process, which the student should undergo in the process of becoming a doctor. It was this piece which alerted me to invert Hunter's phrase, since here the 'necessary humanity' discussed above reasserts itself in a dream. The removal of his clothes is a significant step in Tubby's recognition of his own kinship with the dead. The Chairman's public assessment of Tubby's character and dissection room behaviour is affectionately critical, and, since he is the dissection room skeleton, the Chairman will continue to observe the students, and report back annually to the assembled dead. His is the all-seeing eye of conscience.

Tubby's reciprocal invitation to the dead to join the students' own social gatherings signifies a form of fictive recognition that students who have been through the dissection room will always carry the dissected dead somewhere in their memory, and that some sort of reciprocation will always be due.

For contemporary student readers, a return to the old ways of (mis)behaviour in the dissecting-room may have proved uncomfortable after having read this moral mortal tale. This may indeed have been the writer's intention.

Commentary

A   Now Myddelton Square, Islington, about a mile north of St Bartholomew's Hospital.

B   The fear is of failure in the second pre-clinical exams in anatomy and physiology of the Conjoint Board of the Royal Colleges of Surgeons and Physicians.

C   The Alhambra was a famous Victorian entertainment venue, built in an extravagant Moorish style on the eastern side of Leicester Square.

D   The attempt to know apart the seven carpal bones, which form the wrist, is an age-old problem. An anatomy teacher told one of us that as a student he was tested by having to name them one by one as he spat each bone out of his mouth.

E   The trap door resembled those for barrels over public house cellars. At Bart's, it led down to the corpse reception and preserving room.

F Tubby has adopted anatomists' jargon for dead bodies. Lithotomy position was undignified: individuals were bound by each wrist to each ankle.[25] Corpses were evidently used at Bart's in this era to demonstrate operative procedures.

G In the 1890s all the bodies dissected in medical schools were those of people who had died in workhouses and other institutions housing the poor: those too poor to pay for a funeral. Many dying in such tragic circumstances were elderly. It is unclear in the story why all of them are male, unless it be that the author thought the idea of mixed nudity, even among the dead, would have been too shocking for contemporary readers. Women's bodies were certainly dissected at Bart's at this time.

H Scarpa's triangle, now known as the femoral triangle, is bounded by the inguinal ligament, the medial border of sartorius, and the lateral border of adductor longus.

I Dissection rooms were designed to be cold, to inhibit decomposition. The smells, of preservatives and of the bodies, also meant that ventilation was needed, and the Victorians often used fires to promote air circulation, which of course resulted in draughts. The fires may also have been used to heat water, for the cleaning of bony specimens. In the mid 1920s, there were two fires in the great dissecting room at Bart's, one at each end. They were a favourite gathering point for the students, who got bitterly cold at their work.

J The notion of a conformist revealing his character by stripping off is very wry. The prosector at Bart's prepared dissections, preserved specimens for teaching purposes, and controlled the museum. His room was just along the corridor.

K We find delightful the oblique ridicule of Victorian notions of conformity and the conventions of sociability by their replication here in nudity.

L The notion of sociable gatherings of the dead is more usually associated with Halloween, the old All Hallows Eve (31st October) and the days following. The best known modern survival of this belief is probably the Mexican Day of the Dead.[26] The gathering at Bart's puts us in mind of the more recent practice of thanksgiving services in medical schools for those who have bequeathed their bodies for dissection.[27]

M Cremation was a 'new' form of disposal in the 1890s, and much in the news. The debaters are concerned about physical obliteration.

N The Chairman reveals an awareness that many of those dissected originated from among the uneducated poor. The text makes clear that at least one of the company had been hanged at Newgate: 'I departed my former life amid all the pomp and buffoonery of a death at the nation's expense.' The gallows had been the only legal source of bodies for dissection prior to 1832.[28]

O The cheers for the Chairman's comment here cast the dead as a community keen to assist in the acquisition of medical knowledge.

P The naming procedure described here is akin to that of the medical museum, where specimens are anonymized, and interest focuses upon the medical complaints they exemplify.

Q The dissected dead are portrayed as perceiving dissection as preferable to burial.

Dissection is portrayed as conferring a utilitarian afterlife both in the form of medical knowledge, and as museum specimens. In their last song the dead proclaim themselves as 'men of many parts'.

R   The tune is from the famous music-hall song 'The Man Who Broke the Bank at Monte Carlo'. The words are innocuous when compared with dissecting room ballads memorized by a medical student from his all-male contemporaries at Dublin in the early part of this century, more appropriate to the shower room of a rugby club.[29]

S   The medical pecking order within the institution is very evident.

T   The recognition of continuing relationship between the dead and the students this invitation bespeaks is addressed in our discussion.

U   Mr J— is, as yet, unidentified.

V   As in many folk tales, the stroke of midnight is the cue for spirits to depart. The author is at pains to stress the humanity and normality of the dead.

W   The dead are credited here with institutional loyalty akin to that which students often feel towards their *alma mater*.

X   The idea of haunting offers an affectionate gloss on the relationship between the living and the dead – as though the entire notion of ghosts should be taken as a piece of fun.

Y   The core of the entire text. Reading behind these words, we can see that the story gives a modern medical twist to the older tradition of the cautionary tale. The moral is imparted with a light touch, and with humour.

Notes and references

1   Hunter W. *Introductory lecture to students* c.1780. St Thomas's Hospital Manuscript 55:182. Dr Marion Bowman kindly brought this manuscript to my attention.

2   My informant currently wishes to remain anonymous.

3   Rogers J. *Reminiscences of a workhouse medical officer*. Fisher Unwin: London, 1889.

4   Richardson R, Hurwitz B. Dr Joseph Rogers and the reform of workhouse medicine. *BMJ* 1989;509:1507–10.

5   Lancet sanitary commission on the workhouse infirmaries of London. *Report*. London: The Lancet, 1866.

6   Callaghan D, Ryan C. Ministers in £114m u-turn on GP drugs cash crisis. *Pulse* 2000 Jan 8;**60(1)**:1.

7   Rowlandson T. *Transplanting of teeth*. London: W. Holland, 1790 (Prints and Drawings Department of the British Museum, London). See also: George MD. *Catalogue of personal and political satires in the Prints and Drawings Department of the British Museum*. London: British Museum, 1952;6:744.

8   Richardson R. Transplanting teeth; reflections on a cartoon by Thomas Rowlandson. *The Lancet* 1999;354:1740.

9   Anon [Scott H]. *Adventures of a rupee*. London: J Murray, 1782.

10 Watson W. An account of a disease occasioned by transplanting a tooth. *Medical Transactions of the College of Physicians* 1785;**3**:325–338.

11 Hunter J. *The natural history of human teeth*. London: J Johnson, 1771.

12 David Hamilton's history of tissue transplantation (forthcoming from the OUP) will tell the story in greater depth.

13 Richardson R. *Death, dissection and the destitute*. Chicago: Chicago University Press, 2001.

14 Richardson R, Hurwitz B. Donors' attitudes towards body donation for dissection. *The Lancet* 1995:**346**;277–279. See also: Hurwitz B, Richardson R. Profile of whole-body donors for dissection. *Clinical Anatomy* 1996:**9**;418–9.

15 Bristol Royal Infirmary Inquiry. Interim report: removal and retention of human material. May 2000. The inquiry's web address is www.bristol-inquiry.org.uk See also: Dyer C. Doctors' arrogance blamed for retention of children's organs. *BMJ* 2000:**320**;1359.

16 Royal College of Surgeons of England. *Descriptive catalogue of the pathological series of the Hunterian Museum*. London: RCS, 1966. See also reference thirteen.

17 Wildgoose J. An acceptable body of work? *Daily Telegraph Arts & Books* section 1998 May 5th :Sect A:7. See also: Wildgoose J. Catalogue AN Kelly's exhibition *Birthdays*. London: 291 Gallery, 1999.

18 Richardson R, Hurwitz B. Celebrating New Year in Bart's dissecting room. *Clinical Anatomy* 1996:**9**;408–13.

19 Richardson R. Education and debate: 'a necessary Inhumanity'? *J Med Ethics: Medical Humanities* 2000:**26**;104–6.

20 An earlier version of this piece was published in the journal *Clinical Anatomy*. (Richardson R, Hurwitz B. Celebrating New Year in Bart's dissecting room. *Clinical Anatomy* 1996:**9**;408–13. © 1996 Wiley-Liss, Inc.) It is reprinted here by permission of Wiley-Liss, Inc., a subsidiary of John Wiley & Sons, Inc.

21 Hafferty FW. *Into the valley: death and the socialization of medical students*. New Haven: Yale University Press, 1991.

22 Horne DJ, Tiller JWG, Eizenberg N, Tashevska M. Reactions of first-year medical students to their initial encounter with a cadaver in the dissecting room. *Academic Medicine* 1990:**65**;645–6.

23 Gustavson N. The effect of human dissection on first-year students and the implications for the doctor-patient relationship. *J Med Ed* 1988:**63**;62–4.

24 Sanner MA. Encountering the dead body: experiences of medical students in their anatomy and pathology training. *Omega* 1997:**35(2)**;173–191.

25 Ellis H. *The history of the bladder stone*. Oxford: OUP, 1969.

26 Carmichael E, Sayer C. *The skeleton at the feast*. London: British Museum Press, 1991.

27 Moreno J. Knowledge and human dignity. *Precepts* (State University of New York Health Science Newsletter) Brooklyn, NY: 1991:**3(2)**;1–5.

28 See reference 13.

29 Smith D. *Dissecting room ballads*. Dublin: Black Cat Press, 1984.

CHAPTER TEN

On interpretation

Jonathan Glover

What have paintings and novels, poems and plays, to do with medical practice? There is no single answer. Different people will take away different things from a novel. Some may not be affected at all. And of those who are changed a bit by reading it, not all will be changed in the same way. If there is a single 'message' to be taken away, it is a rather crude novel. And even less are there simple messages to be taken away from literature or the arts as a whole.

All the same, people often *are* changed and enriched by the arts, and sometimes in ways that bear on being a good doctor. Here I want to take one aspect of the arts – mainly literature – that may help shape a doctor's approach. A central theme of so much art, particularly painting and literature, is the interpretation of people.

A doctor has to do a good deal of interpretation. This is partly because we patients are fairly inarticulate when it comes to saying what is wrong with us. Virginia Woolf once said that 'the merest schoolgirl who falls in love has Shakespeare and all the poets to speak for her', but when she goes to the doctor she has no-one to help her describe her pain. We patients often feel baffled when asked what kind of pain we feel and so the doctor has to interpret our vague replies, our 'crudest grunts and noises'.[1] And this requires getting an impression of what we are like, in order to distinguish between our usual characteristics and features of the illness. A general practitioner once told me that a doctor's own response to someone is often the most sensitive medical instrument.

We all know that in much illness there is a psychological component. I have always admired John Berger's book *A fortunate man*[2]. It is about a country doctor who starts with a purely physiological approach to illness, but over time comes to see that illness is sometimes linked with the history of a patient's whole personality. This is a key insight. Illness may be caused entirely by mechanical failure, but often these things are interwoven with psychology. Tracy's striking phrase that she does not want to be seen as an 'illness with a person attached'[3] provides a timely reminder of the importance placed by patients on a medical appreciation of their psychological as well as their physical needs.

In psychiatry, interpretation is of particular importance. Psychiatrists, like all of us, have to 'read' other people's behaviour, to see that someone is not waving but drowning. Because psychiatry is under-funded, interpretation is sometimes played down. Psychotherapy is expensive compared to medication. But even pharmacological treatment requires interpreting the patient.

The bizarre behaviour of people with major psychiatric illness often makes them extremely difficult to interpret. Some of the great nineteenth and early twentieth century psychiatrists admitted that they did not always succeed in their attempts at intuitive understanding. Eugen Bleuler said that people with schizophrenia seemed to him stranger than the birds in his garden. Karl Jaspers, perhaps the greatest philosophical psychiatrist, said it was possible to have empathy for those with mood disorders but not for those with schizophrenia. Faced with such people we feel a gulf that defies description.[4]

The growth of biological psychiatry has produced treatments of immense benefit. In defending a humanistic approach to psychiatry, I am in no way arguing against a biological approach. This is one of the fields where humanism and science, far from being incompatible, are both essential. It is a terrible thing to have schizophrenia now, but it was far worse before current drug treatments. Because of the relative success of biological psychiatry, it is tempting to think that is the only way that the future should go. But we also need to develop, as far as we can, ways of trying to decode the human meaning of what psychiatric patients do and say, so that they do not seem stranger than the birds in the garden.

One approach is that of the psychiatrist Louis Sass, who has been struck by the fact, embarrassing to people in my profession (teachers of philosophy), that a lot of what philosophers talk about is what psychiatric patients talk about too.[5]

In an academic context, philosophers discuss such questions as 'How do I know there is a world outside my mind?', 'How do I know other people are conscious?' or 'Someone may look just like the person I met yesterday, but how do I know that they really are the same person?' It is salutary to be reminded that these are often the same issues that obsess many patients in psychiatric hospitals. We philosophers do it as a kind of intellectual game. It is a game with a serious purpose: to get clear about the basis of our everyday knowledge or about the nature of personal identity. But the questions are asked in a hypothetical spirit and normally reflect no personal existential crisis. One way of marking off some psychiatric patients from philosophers is the idea that the patients think about the same questions and doubts, but take them seriously and personally. And perhaps what marks off these patients from most other people is their framework of interpretation. They have the same evidence as the rest of us about what the world is like, but disagree with the conventional interpretation.

Sceptical questions arise in science and in medicine, but they are typically both more localised and more practical than philosophical scepticism. Perhaps a drug used in treating diabetes is supported by poor scientific evidence, or may have previously unnoticed side effects? Such scepticism might lead to greater caution in prescribing the drug, and very likely to research that might settle the questions. But sceptical questions in philosophy, being about the whole framework of our thought, are harder to resolve and have less practical upshot. A philosopher questioning the basis of our belief in physical objects cheerfully uses a computer to type the sceptical article.

This, as Louis Sass has pointed out, has links with some features of psychiatric delusions. One is what is called 'double counting': paranoid patients may say that the nurses are trying to poison them, but will still go off and have lunch. Where they behave in a way so inconsistent with the professed belief, it is tempting to say they do not have the belief. But things may not be so simple. They may still hold the belief, but in some non-literal way, so the links to action are cut, in a way reminiscent of some philosophical positions.

The resemblance to philosophical thinking is only one small aspect of schizophrenia. Much remains to be understood. What matters about Sass's account is that it makes a start on understanding the condition from the inside, looking at how people who have it interpret the world. Such attempts at intuitive understanding are now greatly helped by increasing numbers of first person descriptions of psychiatric illness. Students of psychiatry naturally learn about the relevant genetics and neurochemistry. But a whole dimension of understanding will be missing if they do not also read, for instance, Kay Redfield Jamison's autobiographical account *An unquiet mind.*[6]

In psychiatric practice, there is a danger of paring down the role of interpretation and intuitive understanding. Pharmacological treatment takes up much less psychiatric time, and hence much less money, than psychotherapy. And the pressures towards a largely biological practice are also pressures towards largely biological thinking. Some effects of this are visible in how psychiatric services function. Patients can be moved between wards in a hospital for quite small administrative reasons. When they move they often get different psychiatrists and nurses. That might not matter if psychiatric illness were simply a matter of chemical imbalances needing correction by medication. But it does matter a great deal if psychiatric illness also has a human dimension, if its cure involves building up relationships and trust. Particularly in psychiatry, we lose a lot in playing down the role of interpretation.

I want to try to build some bridges between scientific and humanist approaches to people, starting with the modern scientific account of how we perceive the world. A naïve idea of seeing makes the role of the mind a bit like that of the film in a camera. The film is passive, giving an image that corresponds exactly to the pattern of light that falls on it. On this view of seeing, the mind passively receives an experience that is an exact copy of the world we look at. This passive view is something Karl Popper once called 'the bucket theory of the mind': things simply drop into the mind unanalysed, like drops falling into a bucket.[7]

Psychologists and neuroscientists have shown how far from the truth that account is. Even quite simple kinds of seeing are bound up with interpretation in ways our pre-scientific selves might not appreciate. There are complex and active analysing mechanisms, starting in the retina and going all the way back to the visual cortex. And similar things can be said of hearing and the other senses.

The art historian Ernst Gombrich has discussed how, when we paint or draw, our attempts to reproduce the world are always influenced by a tradition.[8] On my first day at school, I was asked to draw a house. I had seen houses, but I had no clue about how to represent them on paper. So, as any child might, I looked to see what the others were doing, and did that too. Gombrich suggests that much of the history of art is a little like that. He talks about the process of 'schema and correction': in art we start with an idea or stereotype, often derived from others, and then modify it as we develop our own style. He suggests that in painting there is no such thing as the innocent eye.

Seeing itself is like that too. We never look at things with the innocent eye. Instead, in all perception there is a process rightly likened to testing hypotheses: we try out interpretations and discard them if they do not fit. You see a blur in the distance. You look and put forward a hypothesis. Perhaps it is Uncle Jack's car: he said he would arrive about now. Then it comes a bit closer and you are not so sure. It looks a bit grand for Uncle Jack: he has a battered old Mini and this looks now a bit like a Jaguar, so it probably isn't him. We do not just passively see, but actively impose and revise interpretations. In this case we are doing it consciously, but what psychology and neuroscience have started to unravel is how perception which at the conscious level is unproblematic depends on the brain carrying out a very similar process of testing hypotheses below the level of consciousness.

These mechanisms of interpretation can go wrong. Some neurological disorders shed light on the mechanisms in ordinary perception that function without our being aware of them. For instance, people with agnosia see things without recognising them. The core visual system is intact, but the mechanism by which we classify, interpret and recognise is faulty.

As well as interpreting things in general, we particularly interpret people, and especially their faces. The psychologist Nicholas Humphrey has put forward the idea that, on evolutionary grounds, we should not be surprised that we are good at interpreting each other.[9] In the early history of the human race, other people's attitudes of friendship or hostility must often have been crucial for survival. One route to survival might be the development of very powerful intuitive mechanisms for decoding other people's emotional states from their posture, movement, tone of voice and so on. In the neurological condition prosopagnosia, people with particular lesions can recognise everything except faces. This suggests a specific brain mechanism devoted to interpreting faces, which is what would be expected on Humphrey's evolutionary account.

The interpretation of someone's face can also be inseparable from the beliefs we have about them. Marcel Proust's narrator in *Remembrance of things past* makes this point vividly:

> Even the simple act which we describe as 'seeing someone we know' is to some extent an intellectual process. We pack the physical outline of the person we see with all the notions we have already formed about him, and in the total picture of him which we compose in our minds those notions have certainly the principal place. In the end they come to fill out so completely the curve of his cheeks, to follow so exactly the line of his nose, they blend so harmoniously in the sound of his voice as if it were no more than a transparent envelope, that each time we see the face or hear the voice it is these notions which we recognise and to which we listen.

The narrator talks about his parents' friend Swann. One of the narrator's vices is that he is a tremendous snob, so that for him it was a very important fact about Swann that he moved in very exalted social circles when in Paris. But the narrator's parents do not know this about him and so they see a different man: 'from the Swann they had constructed for themselves, my family had left out, in their ignorance, a whole host of details of his life in the world of fashion, details which caused other people, when they met him, to see all the graces enthroned in his face ...'.[10]

Seeing faces involves these complex layers of interpretation. There may be recognition of whose face it is. There may be the ability to read emotions in facial expressions, possibly biologically programmed in part. And the whole process may be coloured by other beliefs we hold about the person.

Perhaps all this contributes to the extraordinary power of the series of self-portraits Rembrandt painted over his lifetime. What makes those paintings great is not just that they are very accurate pictures of what his face was like. You see him first as a supremely confident young man. You also know that it is not the face of just any person, but of Rembrandt, the painter of these astonishing portraits. The young man had something to be confident about. You then follow the face across his life. In the faces of old age, there is reflected both enriched wisdom and an old person's sadness. The sense of human depth that we respond to so much in these self-portraits comes partly from Rembrandt's ability to convey a sense of shared interpretation. He intended his faces to be seen in these ways, and we recognise his intention.

A few years ago, the Hayward Gallery had an exhibition drawn from the Prinzhorn collection of art by psychiatric patients in a German hospital.[11] At about the same time that I visited this exhibition, a friend gave me a book of Van Gogh's self-portraits. I had not looked at these self-portraits since I was a schoolboy, when I had liked them very much and had thought them powerful and strong. But, because the rather common reproduction of Van Gogh's paintings had turned them into a kind of cliché, I had lost interest. Seeing these portraits again, so much later in my life, and with the art of psychiatric patients in mind, I found them almost unbearable to look at. They were tormented in a way I had not understood, and tormented in a distinctively psychiatric way. What is it about the way psychiatric patients see things which has something in common with Van Gogh? If we could understand this (and I have nothing to offer here) we might understand their condition a lot better. Once again, what is needed is not causal explanation but interpretation.

A final word about the role of intuition in interpretation. I want to defend our first, intuitive impressions of people. They are not always right, but we should take them seriously. Ted Hughes, in a talk to children about writing poems, spoke about those first impressions which 'we cannot pin down by more than a tentative vague phrase. That little phrase is like the visible moving fin of a great fish in a dark pool.'[12] We do have a great capacity for intuitive understanding of people. We can often understand people from the inside.

In autism, it looks as if the mechanisms of this intuitive understanding have in some way failed to develop. There is a great debate about whether those who have autism lack a 'theory of mind' for other people, or whether they are not very good at simulating what it is like to be another person. Perhaps these approaches are not entirely distinct. Part of the evidence for the 'simulation' view is that autistic children do not do much pretend play. There might be a link between this and the examples in this book of creative writing stimulating a greater degree of empathy. Pretend play is something children use in learning to develop an understanding of other people, so perhaps this kind of writing is also relevant.

The hope is that the use of the humanities in medical education will encourage empathy. People who read or write novels or poems, or who paint or come to like looking at paintings, may develop and share intuition and empathy. This may contribute something to the appreciation of our shared humanity. Or, if that is a bit grand, there is the more modest thought that some of us would rather be treated by a doctor who is not only an expert on disease, but also has a feel for people.

Notes and references

1   Woolf V. On being ill. In: Bowlby R (ed.). *The crowded dance of modern life.* Middlesex: Penguin, 1993.

2   Berger J, Mohr J. *A fortunate man: the story of a country doctor.* Middlesex: Penguin, 1967.

3   See page 34.

4   Jaspers K. *General psychopathology* (translated by Hoenig J, and Hamilton MW). Baltimore: John Hopkins University Press, 1997.

5   Sass LA. *The paradoxes of delusion: Wittgenstein, Schreber and the schizophrenic mind.* Ithaca: Cornell University Press, 1994.

6   Jamison KR. *An unquiet mind: a memoir of moods and madness.* New York: Alfred A. Knopf Inc., 1995.

7   Popper K. *Objective knowledge: an evolutionary approach.* Oxford: Oxford University Press, 1972.

8   Gombrich EH. *Art and illusion.* London: Phaidon Press, 1960.

9   Nicholas Humphrey: *The inner eye.* London: Faber and Faber, 1986.

10 Marcel Proust. *Remembrance of things past* (translated by Scott-Moncrieff CK, Kilmartin T). London: Chatto & Windus, 1981.

11 *Beyond reason: art and psychosis; works from the Prinzhorn collection.* London: Hayward Gallery, 1997.

12 Hughes T. *Poetry in the making.* London: Faber and Faber, 1967.

Further reading

This reading list has been compiled from the suggestions of contributors to this book. It is by no means exhaustive but is an attempt to share with readers some of the books which others have found thought-provoking and inspiring. Much has been written about the value of literature in enabling practitioner understanding of complex human issues. Some of these texts are referred to below, and these provide valuable insight into the power and potential of the arts in healthcare.

We would encourage readers to view the whole of literature, film and art as an exciting resource for their work and not to feel constrained by lists of so-called appropriate or key works.

Journals

The new BMJ journal, *Medical humanities*, highlights educational initiatives and ideas in this field. International journals include the US publications *Literature and medicine* and *Journal of medical humanities*.

Websites

Syllabi for medical humanities courses across the United States and Canada are available on-line, thanks to a splendid resource run out of New York University (NYU) as part of the *On-line database of literature and medicine (New York University School of Medicine)* which can be accessed at

http://endeavor.med.nyu.edu/lit-med

The Medical Humanities Unit, with advice and support from NYU, is in the process of setting up a similar UK-based on-line database of courses offered in the UK which will be available in the near future at

http://www.ucl.ac.uk/primcare-popsci/mhu/conference.html

The arts and medicine: general works

Cassell EJ. *The place of the humanities in medicine*. Hastings on Hudson, New York: The Hastings Centre, 1984.

Cassell, EJ. *The nature of suffering and the goals of medicine*. Oxford: OUP, 1991.

Downie RS (ed.) *The healing arts: an anthology*. Oxford: OUP, 1994.

Evans, M, Sweeney K. *The human side of medicine*. London: RCGP (Occasional Paper 76), 1998.

Haldane D, Loppert S. (eds). *The arts in health care: learning from experience*. London: King's Fund Publications, 1999.

Morris D. *Illness and culture in the postmodern age*. London: University of California Press, 1998.

Philipp R, Baum M, Mawson A, Calman K. *Humanities in medicine: beyond the millennium*. London: Nuffield Trust, 2000.

Ratzan RM, Carmichael A (eds.). *Medicine: a treasury of art and literature*. Beaux Arts Editions, 1991.

The role of narrative in medicine

Brody H. *Stories of sickness*. New Haven, CT: Yale University Press, 1987.

Broom B. *Somatic illness and the patient's other story*. London: Free Association, 1997.

Campo R. *The desire to heal – a doctor's education in empathy, identity and poetry*. London: WW Norton, 1997.

Greenhalgh T, Hurwitz B (eds.). *Narrative based medicine*. London: BMJ Publishing, 1998.

Montgomery Hunter K. *Doctors' stories: the narrative structure of medical knowledge*. Princeton, NJ: Princeton University Press, 1991.

Sontag S. *Illness as metaphor*. London: Allen Lane, 1979.

Walker S, Rosfman R (eds) *Life on the line: selections on words and healing*. Mobile, AL: Negative Capability Press, 1992.

Books about therapies involving the arts

Bolton G. *The therapeutic potential of creative writing; writing myself.* London: Jessica Kingsley, 1999.

Connell C. *Something understood: art therapy in cancer care.* London: Wrexham Publications, 1998.

Patient perspectives

Diamond J. *C: Because cowards get cancer too.* London: Vermillion, 1999.

Harris M. *Odd man out.* London: Pavilion Books Ltd, 1996.

Picardie R. *Before I say goodbye.* Middlesex: Penguin, 1998.

Zola I. *Ordinary lives: voices of disability and disease.* Cambridge: Applewood Books, 1982.

Brighton J, Savage A (eds). *The patient knows.* Cardiff: Marches Cancer Care, 1997.

The carer's perspective

Loader J (ed). *Cold comfort.* London: Serpent's Tail, 1996.

Martz S (ed). *If I had my life over I would pick more daisies.* Watsonville, CA: Papier Maché Press, 1992.

Spark D. *Last things.* Boston: Ploughshares, 1994.

The doctor as patient

Vaughan C. Teach me to hear mermaids singing. *BMJ* 1996;**313**:565.

Wyoka J. Hospice at Home. *BMJ* 1995;**311**:1687–8.

The doctor's perspective

Berger J, Mohr J. *A fortunate man: the story of a country doctor.* Middlesex: Penguin, 1967.

Selzer R. *Letters to a young doctor.* New York: Touchstone, 1982.

Singh S. Around every tumour there's a person. *BMJ* 1996;**316**:560.

Illness, patients and doctors in fiction

de Bernieres L. *Captain Corelli's mandolin*. London: Minerva, 1995.

Flaubert G. *Madame Bovary*. Middlesex: Penguin, 1950.

Holman S. *The dress lodger*. London: Sceptre, 2000.

Solzhenitsyn A. *Cancer ward*. Middlesex: Penguin, 1971.

Stevenson RL. *Dr Jekyll and Mr Hyde*. Middlesex: Penguin, 1979.

Welsh I. *Trainspotting*. London: Secker & Warburg, 1993.

Informative texts in humanites subjects relevant to this field

Glover J. *A moral history of the twentieth century*. Jonathan Cape: London, 1999.

Porter R (ed). *The Cambridge illustrated history of medicine*. Cambridge: CUP, 1996.

Porter R. *The greatest benefit to mankind: a medical history of humanity from antiquity to the present*. London: Fontana Press, 1997.

Richardson R. *Death, dissection and the destitute*. Chicago: University of Chicago Press, 2001.

Scheme of modules for the MA (Wales) in Medical Humanities

University of Wales, Swansea

This is a curriculum, showing typical selected topics in each module. The precise selection of topics varies slightly from year to year.

Module 1: Models of mankind and medicine
- ▶ Cultural versus technological approaches to medicine and health care
- ▶ Wholeness, healing, health; conceptions of illness and disease
- ▶ The mind/body problem
- ▶ Biological life and biographical life (bodies and persons)
- ▶ The goals of medicine; the practice of clinical medicine as an art and as a science

Module 2: Sociology and anthropology of medicine and health care
- ▶ Lay constructions of health and illness
- ▶ Orthodox medicine and the organisation of health care
- ▶ Alternative systems of medicine and healing
- ▶ The health care professions
- ▶ Cultural understandings of death

Module 3: Social history and politics of medicine and health care
- ▶ The development of hospital medicine and general practice in Britain
- ▶ The development and nature of public health
- ▶ Institutional care versus 'community' care
- ▶ Technological and population changes: their impact on work and health
- ▶ World health: geopolitical boundaries and moral responsibilities

Module 4: Medicine, health care, literature and the arts
- ▶ The role of metaphor and narrative in clinical understanding
- ▶ Narratives of illness and medicine in the novel and poetry
- ▶ Health and illness as subject and metaphor
- ▶ Visual images and the representation of illness and medicine
- ▶ The photograph as a document

Module 5: Medicine, health care and religion
- ▶ Relations between religion and science
- ▶ Suffering and meaning
- ▶ Religious roots of medicine and health care
- ▶ Medical accounts of religious belief
- ▶ Religious and other accounts of healing

Scheme of modules for the BSc in Medical Sciences and Humanities
University of Wales, Swansea

The degree in Medical Sciences and Humanities involves the pursuit of six strands of study over three years. Three of the strands are science – and three are humanities-based. The content of the strands is given in more detail in the table below. In the final year students must complete a project on a subject of special interest.

	Year 1	Year 2	Year 3
Strand A			
Biological sciences	Genetics and microbiology / Cell biology and histology	Human anatomy and physiology / Biochemistry of biological systems	Pharmacology / Biochemistry of neurones
Strand B			
Physical sciences: chemistry	Foundational, introductory and general chemistry	Foundations of organic chemistry	Human chemistry
Physical sciences: physics	Mechanics and hydrodynamics	Electricity and magnetism	Physics of the body
Strand C			
Clinical sciences	Acquiring information in medicine / Introduction to psychology in medicine	Appraising information in medicine / Administration of health care	Applying information in medicine / Public health medicine

Appendix B *continued*

	Year 1		Year 2		Year 3	
Strand D						
Philosophy of medicine	Introduction to philosophy of medicine	Medicine, science and values	Health, disease and illness	People, populations and medical care	Persons and illness	*Free-standing project*
Strand E						
Social sciences and medicine	Medicine and society	Introduction to health economics	Sociology of medicine		Health policy	
Strand F						
Literature and medicine		Introduction to literature and medicine		Medicine and literature: Romantic poetry		Medicine and literature: Modernist prose
History and medicine	Introducing medical history		Medicine, politics and public health		The development of hospital medicine	

Index